Backache:
its Evolution and
Conservative Treatment

Backache:
its Evolution and
Conservative Treatment

David P. Evans
MSc (Biomechanics), MD

Department of Rheumatology
University Hospital of Wales
Cardiff

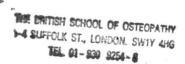
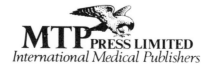

MTP PRESS LIMITED
International Medical Publishers

Published by
MTP Press Limited
Falcon House
Lancaster, England

Copyright © 1982 David P. Evans

First published 1982

British Library Cataloguing in Publication Data

Evans, David
  Backache: its evolution and conservative treatment.
  1. Backache
  I. Title
  616.7′3   RD738

  ISBN 0–85200–430–3

Phototypesetting by Swiftpages Ltd, Liverpool and
printed by Butler & Tanner Ltd, Frome and London

Contents

Part 3 Conservative Treatment of the Abnormal Back

Introduction

Backache is a frustrating symptom even to those practitioners who specialize in locomotor medicine because of the inability in most cases to arrive at a precise diagnosis. This leads to uncertainty about the best method of treatment likely to help the patient. Much of the confusion arises from misunderstandings concerning the nature of back pain and misconceptions abound. The first of these misconceptions is the belief that the spine in man is solely a supporting pillar. Its role in locomotion is neglected. Yet it is the very flexibility allowing locomotion which, when abused, leads to many of the causes of backache. The second misconception is the belief that man has back problems simply because he stands on his hindlegs in an erect posture. A study of evolution shows us that man has been erect for at least five million years but probably only plagued by backache in the last 10 000 years – a time that corresponds to his habit of picking things up and carrying them around. Picking up an object, even when done properly with a straight back and flexed knees, is not the only problem. Equal damage is done when we find where to put the object and rotate in order to put it down. A third misconception, therefore, is that it is only lifting heavy objects that leads to trouble. Rotating with light, awkward loads can be equally hazardous.

The whole subject is fraught with myth and dogma, so we must go back to the very beginning and examine the evolution of the spine to try and find a pathway leading to a rational basis for conservative treatment. In this monograph the chapters are linked by a logical progression of concepts and these are listed in order at the end of each chapter. This is to encourage the reader to become conversant with an overall view of the biomechanics of backache rather than use the text as a reference work.

Very few ideas in medicine are original and the contribution of each worker is usually small. My contribution is no exception and lies in the treatment-end of this story where I have tested various treatments advocated for patients suffering from low back pain. I rely heavily on other workers for the remainder of the book but rather than paraphrase their writings I often quote them at length (I hope always with due acknowledgement). The originality lies in the specific selection of ideas from several authors and the order of their presentation. I am sure that a completely different story could have been told equally well by quoting from the same authors but by using other parts of their texts. By careful selection, attention to order and by supplying a (very) few missing links the following story has evolved. It traces the function of the spine through to the normal spine in man (Part 1), to the abnormal spine in man (Part 2), and finally to the treatment of the abnormal spine (Part 3).

Part 1
The Normal Back

SECTION I
THE VERTEBRAL
COLUMN

1 The locomotion of fish

Our world began 5000 million years ago but life did not exist in any form in the first half of this epoch. Even the first three-quarters of the period since life emerged does not contribute to the fossil record unless high-powered microscopes are used on the fine-grained, flint-like substances called cherts. The last quarter of this period (Figure **1.1**), which has lasted for 600 million years, consists of the Paleozoic, Mesozoic and Cenozoic eras and contains the history of life as told by the fossils.

Throughout the ages plants have retained the ability to build up organic compounds from simple elements which they obtain from their surroundings. Animals, on the other hand, depend on organic nutrition so they need both a system for movement and well-developed sense organs to seek out

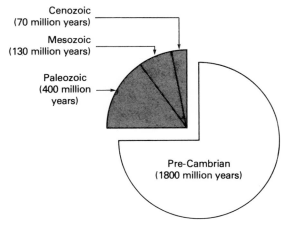

Cenozoic
(70 million years)

Mesozoic
(130 million years)

Paleozoic
(400 million years)

Pre-Cambrian
(1800 million years)

Figure 1.1 Extent of the fossil record

5

their food. During the course of Pre-Cambrian times the first primeval life systems developed into cells and later into multicellular animals and plants. Single-celled organisms, or Protozoa, continued to thrive until the present day using a variety of locomotor mechanisms. Some, like the *Euglena*, gyrate along a spiral path by corkscrew movements of a microscopic lash-like appendage called a flagellum. Others make a tube, or pseudopodium, into which the fluid core of the animal flows. The *Amoeba* is an example of this type of Protozoa and it continually changes its body outline during movement. The Ciliata have more rigid bodies and they are propelled by external delicate hairs which beat in a wave-like motion. Although higher animals have not adopted some of these mechanisms of locomotion, the principles have not been abandoned entirely. Amoeboid movements are characteristic of some white blood cells and the bronchial lining relies on cilia to expel foreign material.

There is a limit to the growth of a single-celled creature, for as size increases the chemical processes inside the cell become difficult and inefficient. Size can be achieved in a different way – by grouping cells together in an organized colony.

Before the Cambrian had reached its half-way mark (Figure **1.2**), sponge-like organisms had built colossal reefs in many parts of the world. The sponges or Parazoa are the most primitive of all multicellular animals and they have survived almost unaltered from the Cambrian to the present day. Sponges show cellular differentiation but there is no cellular specialization into special tissues and organs. They are sedentary animals when adult, and

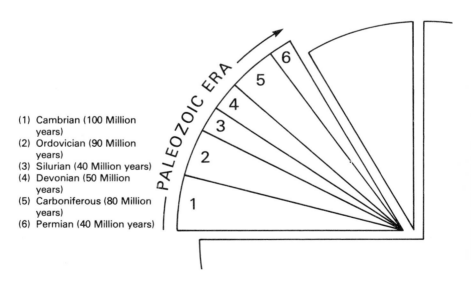

(1) Cambrian (100 Million years)
(2) Ordovician (90 Million years)
(3) Silurian (40 Million years)
(4) Devonian (50 Million years)
(5) Carboniferous (80 Million years)
(6) Permian (40 Million years)

Figure 1.2 The Paleozoic era

if a subkingdom of the animal species remains immobile it must compensate for the ease with which it falls prey to its predators. Sponges have adapted by developing remarkable powers of regeneration to make good the losses which they inevitably incur. Although the scaffolds secreted by the cells form miraculous complexities, sponges can hardly be counted as properly integrated multicellular animals, for without differentiation or cellular specialization they can have no nervous system, no alimentary system and no specific locomotor system.

Fossil examples of all the invertebrate groups are found in deposits of the Cambrian period so all the major animal phyla except the chordates must have developed during the Pre-Cambrian. The first animals with a digestive cavity of sorts were jellyfishes and polyps (the coelenterates). Ancestral flatworms probably developed the first distinct nervous system, and also in the Pre-Cambrian there must have existed an animal from which both the echinoderms and chordates were descended. Metazoa are multicellular animals in which the cells have become organized into groups with differing functions. Some Metazoa change their entire body shape as they move (hydra in the phylum Coelenterata, classes from snails to octopuses in the phylum Mollusca and the phyla containing the flatworms, roundworms and segmented worms), while others maintain a rigid body shape and rely on external appendages for locomotion. The phylum Arthropoda consists of examples of the latter, moving on jointed legs attached to an external or exoskeleton. Soft-bodied invertebrates like segmented worms use a totally different system. These animals neither have a hard external nor internal skeleton but its place is taken by fluid under pressure. This functions as a hydrostatic skeleton and is surrounded by muscles which contract against it. Earthworms and leeches move by alternately contracting longitudinal and circular muscles, the earthworm retaining gained ground with bristles underneath it and the leech with suckers at each end of it. In these animals the longitudinal muscles shorten on the two sides of the body at the same time, whereas in the marine worm *Neresis* the body does not elongate and shorten but bends alternately to one side or the other. The muscles on one side do not shorten simultaneously but in a definite order, throwing the body into a series of curves. The body is covered with many small paddles and the effect of waves travelling throughout the length of the animal propels it through the water.

A distinction is often made between the vertebrates, which comprise only one phylum and include some of the most highly organized representatives of animal life, and the invertebrates which represent all the other animal phyla. It is not appreciated that the various invertebrate phyla are often as distinct one from another as they are from vertebrates. Consequently many phyla among the invertebrates contain representatives that are just as highly organized as are some of the chordates. The insects, for example, are as physiologically complex as mammals although their plan of organization is entirely different. Petersen (1963) reminds us that when we speak of animals as being higher and lower forms, we should bear in mind that these terms have real as well as relative meaning. A descendant form is always higher on the evolutionary time-scale, in other words, it is younger chronologically. However this does not necessarily indicate a higher – in the sense of better – degree of development. Both ancestor and descendant forms are well adapted to a particular environment. Since evolution is a historical process, all that has gone before has to influence what is occurring and will occur.

Compared to the snail-like pace of animal development in the Pre-Cambrian, the first 230 million years of the Paleozoic era, which comprise the Cambrian, Ordovician and Silurian periods, can be regarded as a veritable explosion. This was the Age of the Invertebrates. Geological evidence shows that around the middle of the Cambrian period the oceans began to rise and the land was reduced to groups of very large islands. These islands were completely barren but in the sea life flourished and spread from pole to pole. Every one of the twelve or more great subdivisions of the animal kingdom today has some representatives that live in water whilst only four of the subdivisions have representatives that walk on land. This rather striking fact is further evidence that animal life began in water and that land-living forms evolved at a later date. In water radial symmetry is characteristic of animals which are fixed to the bottom or float about with the currents. Active animals are almost always bilaterally symmetrical and activity is an attribute of vertebrates. Water, particularly sea-water, offers considerably more resistance to objects moving through it than air. Aquatic animals are streamlined in order to minimize this resistance. A study of models of different shapes shows that water can flow most readily over a body shaped rather like a blunt-ended cigar. An animal with this ideal shape has to be endowed with cilia, paddles or some compensatory method of propulsion. Many species, for example, lancelet and fish, are propelled by muscles which act against a rigid internal support so continually modifying their fusiform shape. The first vertebrates probably developed in shallow rivers and inland lakes. Their proficiency at swimming points towards their having evolved in running water, and the oldest traces are found in Ordovician and Silurian deposits which have been interpreted by most authorities as being of freshwater origin. It must have been at a later date that they spread to the oceans although the early stem chordates may have been marine creatures. The fish-like type of locomotion is more effective than that of invertebrates in water and the advantage becomes even greater in running water.

We do not know what the progenitor of the first known vertebrates looked like but there still lives today a semi-transparent little creature that perhaps gives an indication of the appearance of our earliest forebears. This animal, the lancelet, lives on sandy beaches throughout most of the globe. These creatures swim with jerky movements in which the tail is drawn towards the head with lightning speed causing the body to assume an S-shape, and then they straighten up. They repeat this manoeuvre for several seconds making little headway and then fall over on their side as though exhausted. These same movements permit them to burrow into soft, wet sand with surprising speed. The body is practically all trunk and tail, for there is no cephalization. The internal support of the lancelet is a notochord which persists along the whole length of its body throughout life. The interior of this rod is filled with a soft jelly-like substance, which in itself has no strength but it is enclosed in a tough sheath, and the combination of the two makes an excellent support-ing structure which is fairly firm but flexible. The muscles are arranged in clearly marked segments all along both sides of the notochord.

Agnatha are a subphylum of vertebrates characterized by the absence of jaws. They are especially interesting because certain extinct forms are the oldest known vertebrates. These animals, the ostracoderms, lived nearly 500 million years ago. They were slow, bottom-dwelling fish covered with thick plates of bone scales over the trunk and a solid layer of armour plates over the head. The mouth was usually a round sucker-like opening underneath the head end of the animal. They were not predatory but obtained their food from the mud.

Lampreys are present-day Agnatha which still have large buccal funnels lined with horny denticles allowing the adult lamprey to attach itself to its host fish whilst a tongue-like rod rasps the flesh of the victim. The lampreys are amongst the lowliest of living vertebrates but possess the beginnings of a backbone although they lack jaws.

The armoured condition of the early vertebrates has led to the term ostracoderms or shell-skinned. Bone, in the shape of both surface armour and internal skeletal parts, is an extremely old vertebrate characteristic. The sturgeon, with hardly any bone in its body, has descended from forms with a well-ossified skeleton and it is probable that other modern species which have no bones, such as lampreys and sharks, are degenerate rather than primitive types. The earliest fish-like vertebrates with jaws – the placoderms – had appeared by the end of the Silurian period. With the development of the jaw active life off the bottom became possible, and lift and steering were provided by pectoral and pelvic fins. Today cartilaginous fish either use their tail for propulsion with vertical, dorsal fins preventing yawing from side to side and the pectoral fins providing lift (for example sharks) or, if their tail plays little part in the locomotion, they have large pectoral fins which are used in a wave-like flapping motion (for example, rays).

Early placoderms had characteristics pointing both to cartilaginous and bony fish. They may be close to the direct progenitors of both these two groups (Figure **1.3**). The placoderms became extinct at the end of the Permian and the cartilaginous and bony fish appeared at the beginning of the Devonian. Both are independent lineages derived at approximately the same time. The bony fish, from their very beginning, can be divided into

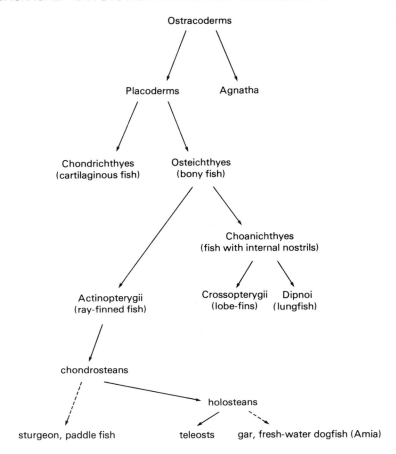

Figure 1.3   The evolution of fish

three main groups: the ray-finned fish, which include the ancestors of the present-day bony fish, the lobe-fins and lungfish. The ray-finned fish can be subdivided into three groups, each one representing a successively higher level of organization. The most advanced grouping are the teleosts which have a completely ossified vertebral column in contrast to the partly cartilaginous one of their forerunners.

Nearly all fish propel the body forwards by use of their tail which moves from side to side in a horizontal plane (Figure **1.4**). In the dogfish the whole of the posterior half of the body moves first to one side and then to the other. This is *carangiform* locomotion. Most other fish use basically the same method of propulsion though different amounts of the body may be involved. In eels the entire body is thrown into lateral undulations which progress from front to rear. This is called *anguilliform* locomotion. There are

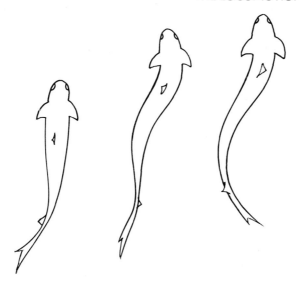

Figure 1.4   Locomotion of a fish

a few fish, for example the trunk fish *Ostracion,* in which propulsion is achieved only by movement of the tail – *ostraciform* locomotion. The movements of the tail result from the shortening and lengthening of muscle fibres lying on both sides of and parallel to the animal's backbone, which with its joints must act as a fulcrum on which the muscles can rock the hinder end of the body and its caudal fin. The backbone has to provide both support for these powerful muscles and be sufficiently pliable to withstand contortion into continually changing sinuous curves. The spine of the fish has to be strong and jointed to fulfil both these criteria. The notochord, although more flexible, was too weak for larger and faster marine forms. Cartilage is also elastic and flexible but its strength makes it an extremely suitable material for all sizes of marine life. Its importance has waned in land animals although its elastic property makes it ideal for the intervertebral discs of man.

It has been accepted generally that the waves of bending observed in swimming vertebrates are produced by contraction on the concave side of each bend of the body at any point within the cycle of movement. Waves of contraction are imagined to pass down the serial myotomes with the velocity of the propagated bends. This interpretation gives no explanation of the source of locomotory thrust or of how the propagation of bends is achieved against external resistance. Blight (1976) has conducted electro-myographic studies in the developmental stage of the palmate newt and in the adult tench. He believes that undulatory propulsion in some animals does not involve waves of contraction, and that the 'waves' recorded in others function in reducing lateral oscillation anteriorly and adapting tail flexibility to different swimming speeds. Swimming of the young newt embryo is accomplished by whip-like behaviour of the tail but the head may swing through as much as 120° in the horizontal plane within the swimming cycle. In early larval life the oscillation of the head is reduced to only a few degrees by the propagation of some kind of 'wave' along the body. This is produced by a delay in myotomal contractions which passes caudally. Violent swimming is accompanied by the return of wide lateral head oscillation. Although waves of contraction are not necessary merely for the propagation of waves of bending, they are also recorded in the adult tench and they require an alternative explanation. The early initiation of contraction on one side of the anterior trunk, while the tail is still moving towards the other side, prevents the full lateral deflection of the head. This reduction of anterior movement may have a hydrodynamic significance, and will certainly have a behavioural significance in stabilizing the cephalic sensory reception during locomotion, particularly in animals which hunt active prey.

Side to side movement of a tail will only result in forward movement if the tail is held in line with the rear end of the body during the power phase from the extreme side position to the midline, whilst during the recoil phase from the midline to the other extreme side position the tail is held at an angle to the body and 'end-on' to the resistance of the water. The tail then realigns with the posterior half of the body and the next power phase is enacted using extremely powerful forces on the fish's tail. The muscles of the trunk enable the trout to produce a thrust equal to at least four times its own weight, accelerating at 45 m/s^2. Fish 'jump' through the water but can only exert these forces for short periods of time. Warm-blooded marine creatures are able to renew their muscular energy much faster than cold-blooded fish. Dolphins can maintain speeds of 30–40 k/h and do not tire anything like so quickly as fish which travel at less than half that speed although they reach their maximum speed in 1/20th of a second.

The bony spine of fish prevents telescoping of the body when the segmental muscles of one side contract. Thus man with his upright stance is not unusual amongst vertebrates in subjecting his spine to compressive forces. The segmental muscles which flex the fish's vertebral axis are attached to ribs as well as to the vertebrae. These costal struts evolved in a dorsal position in the axial musculature in early vertebrates. In fish ventral ribs also appeared, enclosing the caudal vessels within the tail. It is generally agreed that the ribs of land vertebrates correspond to the dorsal series in fish. Ribs are intersegmental in position, and since the basic action of segmental muscles derived from myotomes is to bend the vertebral column, vertebrae are also intersegmental in nature, though their embryonic development shows a primarily segmental pattern. Although there is typically one vertebra per segment, in the tail of *Amia* there are twice as many vertebrae as segments. In lower vertebrates there are dorsal ribs associated with most of the vertebrae, and the vertebrae show little regional adaptation except in the caudal region posterior to the anal opening. As there is no neck in fish, the immediate post-cranial region is able to be occupied by the branchial apparatus. The caudal shift of the respiratory apparatus in land vertebrates was a necessary precursor to the development of a neck, and the ribs became adapted to respiratory function as the limbs took over the responsibility of locomotion from the axial skeleton.

IN SUMMARY

1. Some form of skeleton (exo, endo or hydrostatic) is necessary for locomotion.
2. Active aquatic animals need to be streamlined and symmetrical – so the fusiform shape developed.
3. The need for both a skeleton and a fusiform shape led to the development of an internal longitudinal structure for muscle attachment – the spine.
4. The spine is therefore a locomotor structure which in fish has to undergo side to side undulations throughout its length.
5. A notochord is flexible but not sufficiently strong to resist the compressive forces occurring in larger marine animals so a stronger spine developed – cartilage or bone.
6. Cartilage can withstand the compressive forces even in large fish and, being lighter than bone, it is well suited to form this internal support.
7. The bony or cartilaginous spine had to remain pliable – so it became jointed.

2 The escape from the seas

Vertebrates first set foot on land about 350 million years ago in the Devonian period. At that time the climatic conditions consisted of violent alternations of rainy seasons and severe droughts. The water in the streams and ponds often became stagnant and lacked the necessary oxygen for water-breathing fish. To compensate for the default of oxygen in the water, the primitive lung evolved enabling these fish to come to the surface, gulp down air and breath atmospheric oxygen. Later in more settled climatic conditions this lung in most fish developed into a hydrostatic organ which enabled the fish to rise and sink in the water. All land vertebrates have arisen from those early fish with internal nostrils, the Choanichthyes. These animals were not successful as fish, remaining today only as lungfish and lobe-finned fish. Like the original land-dwellers, present-day lungfish live in regions subject to seasonal drought. They are elongated and eel-like but the fossil record shows that this is a modern tendency. The earliest lungfish had fins separate from each other with a tail tilting upwards. Later the fins became con-centrated at the caudal end of the body and the tail straightened. The tail subsequently fused with the median fins and the paired fins degenerated leading to an eel-like shape. Lungfish were very much more abundant 350 million years ago and their fossils are often found in the same sort of deposits that contain coelacanths. Attenborough (1979) attributes to those two kinds of fish both the essential abilities that the ancient land-exploring fish must have required – locomotion out of water and air-breathing. But because the bones of their skulls are so different from those of the first fossil amphibians, neither fish can be regarded as the one whose descendants eventually colonized the land permanently. This distinction belongs to the ancestors of today's lobe-finned fish. Their skeletons are like those of primitive amphibians with fleshy fins containing skeletal supports instead of typical legs. However, when the fins of fossil specimens are carefully dissected, the lobes at the base are found to be supported by one stout bone close to the body, two bones joined to it and finally a group of small bones and digits – the pattern found in the limbs of all land vertebrates.

Fish that rest on the sea-bed often keep the tips of their paired fins in contact with the ground using them as props to prevent themselves from rolling over. A few, the mudskipper *Periophthalmus* for example, can even creep out of the water and support the front end of their body on breast fins, and they are able to propel themselves on land for moderate distances by hopping along on their tails and fins. To serve as props the fins must be fairly stiff and tightly braced to the lower surface of the body. The next stage in the development of a standing animal was reached when both pairs of lateral fins were used as lateral props and were strong enough to allow the whole body to be held above the ground. No known land-living fish uses its fins in this way but lungfish often rest with the tips of their fins touching the bed of the streams in which they live. In early land-living fish the ends of the fins in contact with the ground were flattened to spread the weight of the animal over a surface large enough to prevent the fins sinking into the soft mud. Lobe-fins had a well-developed bony skeleton without which life on land would not have been possible because limbs of cartilage would not stand the strain of terrestrial life. In the process of change from water to land types, the two limb girdles have become considerably modified. In fish the shoulder girdle is tightly bound to the head while the pelvic girdle is small and confined to the ventral side of the body without any connection to the backbone. In land animals the shoulder must be freed from the head to permit head movements without the need for shifting the front legs, and since the hindlegs must bear much of the weight of the body they must be connected to the backbone.

Amphibians are the most primitive and earliest known forms of four-legged animals. All land vertebrates have been derived from amphibian stock but today amphibians are represented by three comparatively unimportant orders: the frogs and toads, the salamanders and newts, and some rare worm-like forms. All these are highly specialized and have departed far from the first land-forms although salamanders closely approach the body form and general appearance of the most ancient land-dwellers. The body and tail are elongated, the median fins have disappeared but the tail is flattened and is an effective swimming organ. Although the limbs are freely movable they are small and feeble. During locomotion the body is thrown into sinuous curves to gain ground for the legs on which it is supported, and when moving fast these animals swim on the ground on their bellies with their legs hardly touching it. In effect Evans (1946) has shown they exhibit two separate and distinct types of terrestrial locomotion depending upon their speed. When frightened the rapid locomotion effected by violent wriggling of the body over the ground is aided by mucus secreted by the belly skin. The minor role of the legs in rapid locomotion is clearly illustrated when the animal is forced to move over smoked paper. No definite footprints are seen, but instead the main part of the record consists of large irregular smear marks and a more or less undulating line caused by drag of the body and the tail. The legs move in the same sequence as they would if the animal were actually walking but the tips of the digits only just touch the paper. In contrast to this kind of record is that obtained when the animals move in a slow, deliberate manner. In this second type of loco-motion lateral undulations of the trunk produced by the axial musculature still occur but the legs play an important locomotory role. Under normal conditions the animals may remain inactive for relatively long periods, simply lying on the ground with the legs in whatever position they happened to be at the time.

Among the salamanders, and apparently among many extinct groups as well, there are numerous types which have given up the struggle and have gone back to permanent life in the water. So why was life on land attempted? Air-breathing could be accomplished by surfacing alone; the prey of these animals were fish and as they were large they had no enemies. The answer lies in the complete dessication of some pools in seasonal droughts in the Devonian which allowed only those animals able to cross land to reach water again to survive. Thus, according to Romer (1960), land-limbs were developed to reach water not to leave it. Once the development of limbs had taken place the amphibian might learn to linger near drying pools to devour stranded fish, take to eating insects or later to plants. In primitive amphibians the essential pattern of the limbs found in man was already established and the analogue of every human bone was present in these swamp-dwellers. Most of the changes that have occurred in the last 300 million years have been changes in proportions rather than in the addition of new elements.

By the end of the Paleozoic a change of environments took place. Mountains were formed and with this change in the topography of the land there were related shifts in world climates. Local environment varied from swamps, streams and ponds to dry uplands. In these situations during the Permian period the reptiles, which developed from the primitive amphibian stock during the Carboniferous, began to replace the amphibians although some of the latter were able to hang on successfully well into the Mesozoic era. Reptiles were more fully adapted to life on land because their skin was watertight and, unlike amphibians, they did not need to return to the water to breed. This was accomplished by fertilizing, within the body, a type of egg that could be laid on land. The earliest reptiles are known as cotylosaurs or 'stem reptiles' and the first traces of them are found in deposits formed in the great coal swamps when amphibians were still at their peak of development. A typical stem reptile is Seymouria, looking like a sluggish lizard but much more primitive, with short stubby limbs sprawled

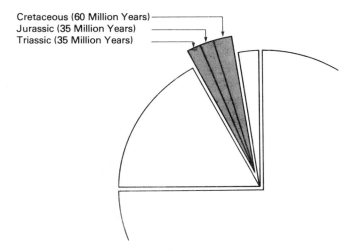

Cretaceous (60 Million Years)
Jurassic (35 Million Years)
Triassic (35 Million Years)

Figure 2.1   The Mesozoic era

out sideways from the body. Then began a great radiation of saurian types which were to dominate the earth during the Age of Reptiles, or Mesozoic era. It began with the close of the Paleozoic era about 200 million years ago and lasted approximately 130 million years. The Mesozoic era is divided into three periods: the Triassic, the Jurassic and the Cretaceous, lasting 35, 35 and 60 million years respectively (Figure **2.1**).

The waddling gait of primitive land-reptiles was clumsy with a broad track and short step. The turtles have retained this old fashioned mode of loco-motion; the lizards have improved their limbs a little but the snakes have abandoned limbs altogether. Several reptilian groups dodged the issue and returned to the water, reshaping their legs into fin-like structures. The reptiles that evolved into mammals remained four-limbed land dwellers but improved their method of walking. A second reptilian group, the archosaurs or ruling reptiles, were the dominant forms on land during the Mesozoic. Speedy locomotion was obtained by running not on all fours but on the hind limbs with the front end of the body lifted from the ground balanced by the long tail. When the burst of speed was over the inefficient front feet were returned to the ground and a four-footed posture was again assumed. In many dinosaurs with a bipedal gait the main reliance was placed on the three centre toes, as the outer one was lost and the inner one often turned back as a rear prop. This arrangement is analogous to the structure of the foot of a bird. During the Cretaceous huge bipeds of the type *Tyrannosaurus* existed with powerful hindlegs but with front ones that had degenerated so much that they were not even able to reach the mouth, much less be useful in walking.

Mammals' ancestors retained all four limbs but rotated them so that the knees were brought underneath the body and the bones of limbs took over most of the strain. Before this adaptation well-developed adductor muscles were necessary to hold the body of primitive tetrapods off the ground, and evidence of the importance of these muscles is shown by the enormous coracoids of the scapulae to which they were attached. These animals expended enormous amounts of energy just to keep their bodies off the ground but in mammals this energy could be used for propulsion. The ancestors of mammals were carnivores leading lives in which a speedy locomotion was necessary. The maintenance of a high body temperature is related to the need of a continuous supply of energy in active animals. The reptilian stem from which mammals sprang was one of the first differentiated from the primitive reptile stock and the first mammals appeared as early as the first dinosaurs. The first stage in the differentiation of mammals from other reptile stocks is that of pelycosaurs, lizard-like carnivores with sprawled-out legs dating back to the late Carboniferous and Lower Permian, a time when the stem reptiles still flourished and ruling reptiles were unknown. The basic placental stock is represented by generalized ancestral insectivores found together with Cretaceous dinosaurs; certain generalized insectivores gave rise to all the other orders of placental animals. These must have begun their differentiation well back in the Cretaceous for at the beginning of the Cenozoic we already find all the major types of placentals in existence. These ancestral placentals looked like shrews in size, outward appearance and general behaviour. They were small and probably shy insectivores, keeping well hidden from the dinosaurs which ruled the earth at that time. A tremendous evolutionary burst occurred in the Cenozoic era which has consequently been called the Age of Mammals. This began about 70 million years ago during a time of continental uplift. The Cenozoic marked the beginning of a long period of mountain-making that is actively continuing at the present day.

IN SUMMARY

8. When aquatic animals rested on land their body required to be supported on fins.
9. The fins were fleshy and developed an internal bony support which in the pelvic region became attached to the backbone to transmit the body weight.
10. The front fins became detached from the head so that the two structures could move independently of each other.
11. The backbone became a strut rather than a compression member and only bony spines were strong enough to fulfil this role. The backbone changed from an organ solely concerned with locomotion to one of support and locomotion.
12. In early land-animals both the backbone and legs were used for

locomotion but in most species (excepting snakes and worm-like amphibians) the legs gradually took over the role. Nevertheless during rapid locomotion the spine resumes responsibility for propulsion of amphibians like the salamander with side to side sinuous movements similar to those of fish.

13. As the backbone is relieved of some locomotor duty it becomes relatively shorter and less flexible but stronger.

14. Some species became bipedal (for example, ruling reptiles) by balancing the body weight with the tail and evolving turned-back toes.

3 The biomechanics of quadrupeds

On land the problem of supporting the body off the ground was not solved easily and the first animals that attempted to overcome the difficulties were not very successful. These early pioneers rested their bellies on the ground in a stance retained by the crocodilians today. Gray (1944) analysed the bending moments along the vertebral column of a series of tetrapod forms

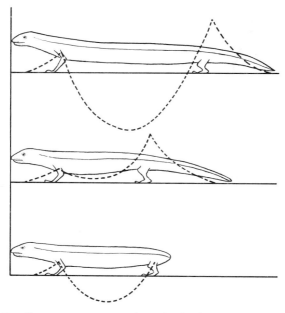

Figure 3.1 Bending-moment curve of vertebral column of various tetrapod forms (after Gray, 1944)

(Figure **3.1**). As the body is shortened the strain on the ventral musculature is lessened. One of the most marked features of later reptilian and early mammalian stocks was a decrease in body length. The effect of the absence of a tail is again to place the ventral musculature under strain. Of interest are the 'sail-bearing' pelycosaurs which exhibited tremendously elongated vertebral spines supporting a sail of skin from the neck to the tail. Both the carnivorous *Dimetrodon* and the herbivorous *Edaphosaurus* were endowed with these odd encumbrances although the former animal was nearly 3 m long. This structure is usually considered to be a temperature regulator by virtue of the large area of skin, well perfused with blood, that can be held either broadside or end-on to the sun. Nevertheless, the shape is closely analogous to that of a bridge constructed as a parabolic girder – an ideal method of spanning a divide between two supporting pillars without placing undue strain on the underside of the beam.

Quadrupeds at once suggest this analogy of two piers supporting a bridge (represented by the forelegs and hindlegs with the weight of the body suspended between). A loaded beam supported at both ends tends to bend into an arc with its lower fibres undergoing a tensile stress and its upper fibres undergoing compression (Figure **3.2**).

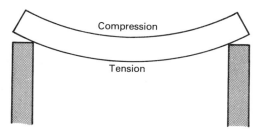

Figure 3.2 A loaded beam supported at both ends tends to bend into an arc with its lower fibres undergoing a tensile stress and its upper fibres undergoing compression

Figure 3.3 Cross-section of girder which has upper and lower flange connected by a web

When the engineer constructs an iron or steel girder he takes advantage of this elementary principle and saves weight by leaving out as far as possible all the middle portion which is the neutral zone, reducing his girder to an upper and lower flange connected by a web (Figure **3.3**).

Ligaments and muscles withstand tensile forces and bones are resistant to compressive forces. We find a paradoxical pattern if we compare a spine to a loaded beam because it appears that the tissues subjected to the tensile forces on the underside of the spine are bone, and the tissue subjected to the compressive forces on the upper side are ligaments (Figure **3.4**). However,

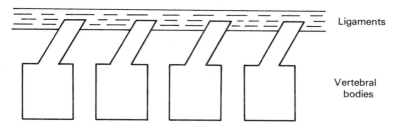

Figure 3.4   Spine of tetrapod showing resistance to tensile forces in upper tissues and resistance to compressive forces in lower tissues

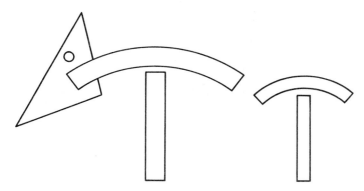

Figure 3.5   Spine of tetrapod represented as two cantilever girders each resting upon its pillar. Now the tensile forces are in the upper fibres and the compressive forces are in the lower fibres

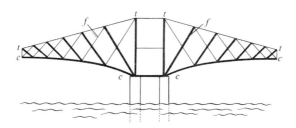

Figure 3.6   Diagram of cantilever girder as used in bridge (after D'Arcy Thompson, 1942)

the configuration can be explained by an alternative system, two cantilever girders each resting upon its pillar (Figure **3.5**).

Now the tensile forces are uppermost and resisted by ligaments and the lower compressive forces are resisted by the vertebral bodies. D'Arcy Thompson (1942) applied strict principles of engineering to the animal's skeleton and described it as beautifully comparable to the main girder of a double-armed cantilever bridge (Figure **3.6**).

The comparative sizes of the two cantilevers varies from animal to animal. In both the horse and the ox the forepart of the animal is much bulkier than its hindquarters and correspondingly the front legs carry more weight than the back legs. Under certain conditions, as when the head is thrust well forward, it is evident that the hindlegs will be relieved of a portion of the

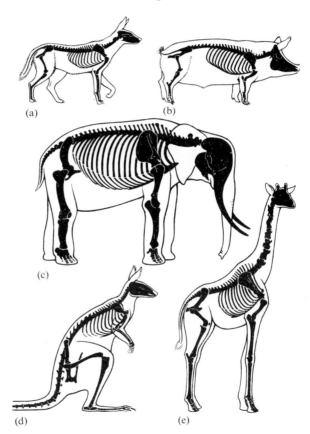

Figure 3.7 Arrangement of the backbone girder in various mammals. (a) Balanced cantilevers (dog); (b) single girder balanced on forelegs and hindlegs (pig); (c) single girder balanced largely about forelegs (elephant); (d) single girder balanced on hind legs (wallaby); (e) single girder balanced on forelegs (giraffe). (from Young, 1975)

comparatively small load which is their normal share. The giraffe represents a single girder balanced almost wholly (and an elephant represents a single girder balanced largely) about the forelegs. The dog has equally balanced cantilevers, while the pig has a single girder balanced on forelegs and hindlegs (Figure **3.7**). Thus the great majority of four-footed terrestrial animals have most of their body weight supported by their forelegs. The chief exceptions are animals with comparatively small heads but large and heavy tails, such as anteaters, kangaroos and dinosaurian reptiles.

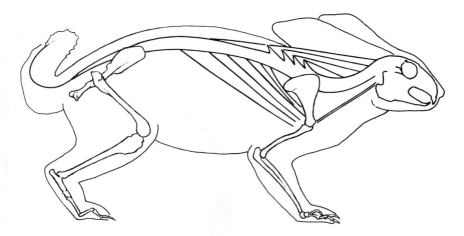

Figure 3.8   Diagram of the skeleton and muscles of the forepart of a rabbit, to show the general arrangement of struts and ties. (after Young, 1975)

In the construction of girders, the depth and hence the strength of the structure should be proportional at every point to the bending moments. For a cantilever system these are greatest at the point of attachment of the support to the girder, and in most quadrupeds the neural spine projecting from each vertebra are largest above the forelegs. The vertebral spines represent the oblique compression members, and the tension members are the ligamentum nuchae beginning along the back of the neck and the various other ligaments and muscles between the vertebral spines. Many other struts and ties are arranged in triangular form and the pattern is shown well in the forepart of the skeleton of a rabbit (Figure **3.8**).

Just as the highest vertebral spines in the horse are those of the withers (the posterior cervical and anterior dorsal vertebrae), a glance at the skeleton of *Stegosaurus* shows the high vertebral spines over the loins, in precise correspondence with the requirements of the bending stress diagram (Figure **3.9**).

In the elephant the dorsal spines are smaller than we might expect

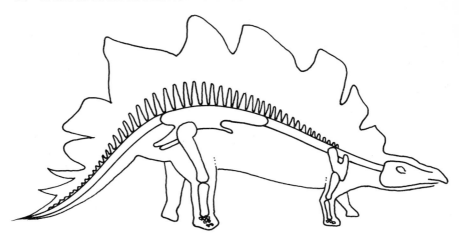

Figure 3.9 *Stegosaurus* showing high vertebral spines over the loins

considering the large forequarters, but in the mammoth, with its immensely heavy and elongated tusks, the bending moments over the forelegs are very severe and the dorsal spines are more conspicuously elevated. In the kangaroo the forelegs are entirely relieved of their load and the spines over the withers are very small. This animal has become bipedal and the lumbar and sacral vertebrae are high and the iliac bones nearly upright. The balance weight of the body is formed by the long, heavy tail which also acts as a third support.

Animals that rest on their hindlimbs have broad feet, the heel rests on the ground and the limbs are relatively short. When the whole sole is applied to the ground the foot is spoken of as plantigrade. Whether an animal is plantigrade or, like the horse, digitigrade, the hindlimb of mammals is usually involved mainly in propulsion and support, and shows less tendency than does the forelimb to modification for special functions. The hip joint is the point about which movements of the body on the hindlegs takes place and the pelvic girdle moves only slightly on the vertebral column. All tetrapod embryos form a pair of ventral cartilaginous pelvic plates which ossify at two centres on each side to form a pubic bone (pubis) anteriorly and an ischium posteriorly. Dorsally on each side an additional cartilage becomes the ilium. At the junction of the three components is the acetabulum, a socket accommodating the head of the femur (Figure **3.10**).

The ilium of tetrapods is firmly ankylosed to the transverse processes of the sacral vertebrae, the site of union being the sacroiliac symphysis. The axial skeleton provides a firm brace against which the femur, now bearing much of the body weight, may push via the pelvic girdle. The two pubic bones typically unite ventrally in a pubic symphysis and the ischia usually form an ischial symphysis. Because of the pubic and ischial symphyses ventrally, and

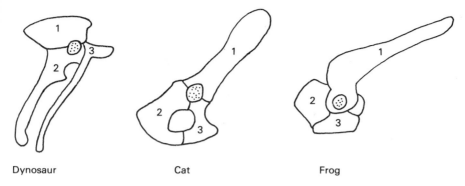

Dynosaur   Cat   Frog

Figure 3.10 Examples of pelvic girdles 1. ilium; 2. ischium; 3. pubis (based on Kent, 1973)

because the ilia are united with the vertebral column dorsally, the caudal end of the coelomic cavity is usually surrounded by a bony ring, the pelvis. The pelvic cavity contains the caudal end of the digestive and urogenital systems. The inferior border of the ring is the pelvic outlet.

In reptiles the ilium is braced against two sacral vertebrae, and it tends to become broader for the attachment of a greater mass of hindlimb muscles, especially in dinosaurs and in lizards that carry the trunk elevated well above the ground. In birds the ilium is greatly expanded to accommodate the musculature necessary for bipedalism and is braced against the lumbar as well as sacral vertebrae. In mammals the ilium, ischium and pubis unite early in postnatal life to form an innominate bone on each side. The two innominates comprise the pelvic girdle and are ankylosed with the sacrum dorsally. The muscles that act at the hip joint have been evolved, like those of the forelimb, within the dorsal (abductor) and ventral (adductor) sheets. A cranioventral group that draws the limb back can be distinguished. In quadrupeds the more caudal braces are especially large and serve to draw the limb caudally, giving the main locomotor thrust. Cranial braces are also prominent and lateral ones prevent the body falling medially. Medial braces prevent the less likely lateral falling. In man the braces all round the joint are important since the balance is likely to be upset in any direction, but the anterior (cranial) and posterior (caudal) braces are especially large.

Apart from the different arrangements of supportive structures, the relative sizes of spines and limbs differ between the species. A horse has comparatively much longer legs than a rat or a lizard. Gray (1959) has shown how short legs and long bodies are adapted for life on steep slopes or on branches of trees whereas the long legs and shorter bodies of horses are adapted for life on relatively flat surfaces. The horse is an example of an animal with its centre of gravity nearer to the forefeet than to the hindfeet, a characteristic of animals which move rapidly. Rabbits, squirrels and bears are examples of animals which stand with their weight held well back towards the hindfeet and consequently either front limb can be lifted from the ground. Some animals bring their centre of gravity so far back that it lies above the hindfeet and the animal becomes bipedal.

Each leg of a walking quadruped is lifted from the ground according to a definite sequence which remains the same throughout all classes of vertebrates. No foot is ever lifted unless the centre of gravity of the body lies over the triangle formed by the other three. As locomotion is quickened, quadrupeds sacrifice the ability to stop at any instant without loss of balance. There are short periods during which only two feet are on the ground. During the gallop of a horse there are periods when no foot is on the ground but the sequence in which the limbs are moved is no longer the same as in walking. The power by which the horse is rapidly driven forwards comes almost entirely from the muscles that move the limbs and relatively little from the muscles of the back. On the other hand, a dog employs lumbar propulsion by alternately flexing and extending its spine during running thus increasing the span between footfalls. The swimming musculature of whales evolved from the non-swimming musculature of terrestrial ancestors. Long antagonistic muscles extend from the whale's skull to the tail and implement the dorsoventral motion, in contrast to the lateral undulations exhibited by fish.

Segmentation is clearly evident in the muscles of the trunk and tail of fish. The body-wall musculature consists of a series of myomeres, or muscle segments, that are separated by connective tissue myosepta. The muscle fibres of each myomere typically arise on one myoseptum and insert into the next. Except in Agnatha the trunk and tail musculature is further divided into dorsal and ventral masses by a horizontal septum that extends between the transverse processes of the vertebrae and the skin. Above the septum are epaxial muscles and below it are hypaxial muscles. Dorsal and ventral sagittal septa separate the muscles of the two sides of the body. In all vertebrates epaxial muscle is typically innervated by the dorsal ramus of the spinal nerve supplying that body segment and hypaxial muscle is innervated by the ventral ramus.

Tetrapods, like fish, exhibit epaxial and hypaxial masses retaining some evidence of their primitive metamerism. Kent (1973) has described adaptive modifications developed as a result of, or associated with, life on land:

(1) The epaxial myomeres have tended to form elongated bundles that extend through many body segments and they have become increasingly buried under the expanding muscles required to operate strong tetrapod limbs. Nevertheless the deepest epaxial muscles still retain their primitive metamerism.

(2) The hypaxial masses have tended to lose their myosepta and to form broad sheets of muscle, especially in the abdominal region. The tendency is

least pronounced in aquatic-tailed amphibians which require segmented muscles for locomotion.

(3) Orientation of the hypaxial musculature into oblique, rectus and transverse bundles has proceeded to a high degree of specialization in tetrapods.

The epaxial muscles of tetrapods lie along the dorsal aspect of the vertebral column in the gutter between the transverse processes and the neural arches. They extend from the base of the skull to the tip of the tail. In urodeles and primitive lizards these epaxial muscles are obviously metameric but in other tetrapods the more superficial epaxial bundles form long muscles occupying several body segments whereas the deepest bundles remain segmental. The longest bundles are the longissimus, iliocostalis and spinalis groups. The shortest bundles are intervertebral muscles that connect one vertebra with the next. The short epaxial muscles in tetrapods perform the same primary function as in fish – producing side to side movement of the vertebral column. Both the short and long bundles of tetrapods can arch the back, a movement most fish cannot perform; the long bundles support the back on land. The extent to which epaxial muscles can bring about these movements depends on the flexibility of the column. In turtles and birds the vertebral column of the trunk is rigid and the associated epaxial muscles are poorly developed, but in the neck and tail the column has movable joints and the muscles are well developed.

The hypaxial muscles of the trunk of tetrapods are divisible into two predominant groups. One group consists of the muscles of the lateral and ventral body walls – the oblique, transverse and rectus muscles, and the other comprises the muscles in the roof of the body cavity forming longitudinal bands on either side of the centra – the subvertebral or hypo-skeletal muscles. The oblique and transverse muscles occupy the lateral body wall and retain their metamerism anteriorly. In modern amniotes, excepting snakes and snake-like lizards, myosepta and ribs have become confined to this anterior part of the trunk (the thorax) and the abdominal wall muscles lack segmentation. The primitive ventrally located rectus bundles of fish have evolved into strong rectus muscles in tetrapods. These help support the ventral body wall where ventral ribs are lacking and also aid in arching the back. In most mammals the rectus extends the entire length of the trunk from the anterior end of the sternum to the pelvic girdle but in man it is confined to the abdominal region. Even in man the rectus muscles are interrupted by narrow myosepta-like tendons reminiscent of myosepta.

The subvertebrals lie immediately underneath and against the transverse processes of the vertebrae. These include the psoas, iliacus and iliopsoas. In the thorax the subvertebrals are less well developed.

The hypaxial muscles of aquatic urodeles are used chiefly for swimming.

Even terrestrial urodeles and limbless tetrapods use them to assist in locomotion. In other tetrapods the total mass of the hypaxial musculature is proportionately reduced because of the shift from locomotion by trunk and tail muscles to locomotion by appendicular muscles. The chief contributions of hypaxial muscles in tetrapods are to support the contents of the abdomen in a muscular sling, to participate in external respiration and to assist the epaxial muscles in bending the vertebral column.

IN SUMMARY

15.   Quadrupeds suggest the analogy of two piers supporting a bridge but examination of the tissues shows compatability nearer a configuration of two balanced cantilevers. The relative size and importance of the two cantilevers differs from species to species, varying through two balanced cantilevers (dog), to a single girder balanced on forelegs and hindlegs (pig), a single girder balanced on hindlegs (wallaby) and a single girder balanced on forelegs (giraffe).

16.   The length of the vertebral spines corresponds with the requirements of the bending stress diagram because these spines are the oblique compression members. They are elongated in the appropriate segment to form the attachment for ligaments and muscles which are under tension.

17.   The hindlimbs of tetrapods are usually involved in both propulsion and support, showing less tendency than does the forelimb to modification for special purposes. Not only is the pelvis always attached to the spine, but the component parts are readily comparable in widely differing species.

18.   The horse, adapted for life on flat surfaces, has a relatively short trunk but long limbs which take over almost entirely the responsibility for locomotion. Some other mammalian groups, for example dogs and the great cats, employ lumbar propulsion. During running they flex and extend their spines thereby increasing the span between footfalls.

19.   Despite the variation between land-vertebrate forms, the trunk muscle masses are divided in the same way into dorsal, epaxial groups and ventral, hypaxial groups. The epaxial myomeres have superficial elongated bundles and deeper bundles which still retain their primitive metamerism.

4

From four legs to two

An animal can only stand on an inclined surface if a vertical line through the centre of gravity passes through the quadrilateral formed by its feet. In practice animals adopt one of two characteristic postures to keep the line of the centre of gravity within this boundary. Either the axes of the limbs are retracted while that of the body is parallel to the slope, or the axis of the body

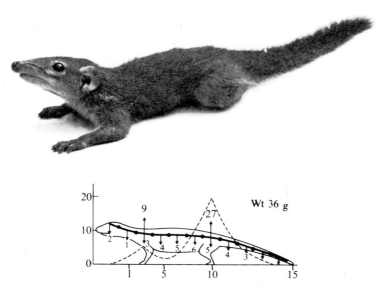

Figure 4.1 The shape of the tree-shrew conforms well to Gray's optimal tetrapod form (after Gray, 1944)

31

is held horizontal by flexure of either the front or hindlimbs. The ancestors of primates were small tree-shrew-like animals with long bodies and short legs so the centre of gravity fell within the pedal quadrilateral on all but the steepest slopes. Although the gravitational effect on their light bodies was of lesser importance than that on larger animals, the strain on the central part of the back and belly was relieved by loading the body weight on balanced cantilevers. The shape of a tree-shrew conforms well to Gray's optimal tetrapod form (Figure **4.1**).

True primates appeared in the middle Paleocene times (Figure **4.2**) and must have been transitional between insectivores and lemurs. Lemurs are typically small and of rather squirrel-like appearance. They are arboreal, nocturnal in habit and the eyes are directed more laterally than forwards. The limbs are moderately long, as is the tail although it is not prehensile. Lemurs are exceedingly primitive primates appearing in the Eocene epoch with the second primate group, the tarsiers. Tarsiers are small, hopping, rat-like creatures surviving today as nocturnal tree-dwellers. They occupy an intermediate position between the lemurs and the third primate group, the anthropoids. The eyes of tarsiers are exceptionally large and are turned completely forward from the primitive lateral position. The orbits are close together above the nose and the two fields of vision are identical. It is now generally felt that the tarsiers are a specialized side-branch of the evolutionary tree, paralleling certain advanced primate developments rather than being true connecting links.

The third and highest division of the primate group are the anthropoids

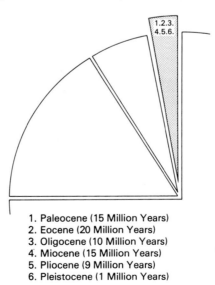

1. Paleocene (15 Million Years)
2. Eocene (20 Million Years)
3. Oligocene (10 Million Years)
4. Miocene (15 Million Years)
5. Pliocene (9 Million Years)
6. Pleistocene (1 Million Years)

Figure 4.2   The Cenozoic era

comprising monkeys, apes and man. No traces of true monkeys are found from before the Oligocene, as the arboreal habits of primates make them notoriously poor items in all fossil collections. All of the anthropoids can sit upright, leaving the hands free for manipulating objects. Flexibility is necessary for climbing trees and there is none of the restriction of limb movement to one plane found in ungulate groups. Although the front limbs are adapted for grasping, four-footed locomotion is still the rule among primates. In some monkeys the tail has developed a prehensile power but in most it is used only as a balancer. Locomotion in the tree has left the skeleton of the primates in a condition much closer to that of the primitive placentals than is the case in most groups. In primitive mammals the thumb and big toes were presumably divergent and this grasping characteristic has in general been retained and emphasized in primates.

Thus tarsiers and anthropoids have evolved two characteristics that have made life in the trees possible – the ability to judge distances by sight, and prehensile hands. In anthropoids the muzzle has retreated and the eyes are close together and directed forward. Only when the two eyes are focused together does depth perception, or stereoscopic vision, become possible. Jumping from branch to branch needs daylight to take advantage of good vision, so we find that all anthropoids (except the douracouli) are diurnal. The perfection of vision has been important in the evolution of the primate brain and is linked with the remarkable degree of intelligence shown by all the anthropoids.

Anthropoids are divided into three groups: ceboids (South American monkeys), cercopithecoids (Old World monkeys) and hominoids (apes and man). Hominoids are divided further into arboreal gibbons and orang-utans, semi-arboreal gorillas and chimpanzees, and man (Figure **4.3**).

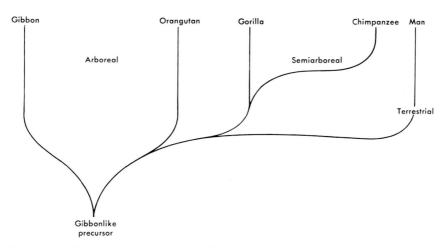

Figure 4.3 Theoretical relationships of hominoids (from Kent, 1973)

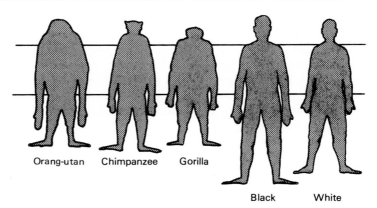

Orang-utan   Chimpanzee   Gorilla   Black   White

Figure 4.4 The proportionate differences between man and the great apes (after Schultz, 1950)

During the transition from the early primates to larger, more recent anthropoids, the trunk has become relatively shorter and the limbs relatively longer. With increasing size, four-footed running along a single branch becomes increasingly difficult. The weight can be distributed if the animal rests his feet on one branch and grasps an overlying one with his arms. From this it is but a step to the type of locomotion in which true brachiators, gibbons and orang-utans, are adept. These apes swing by the hands from bough to bough and the arms are much elongated. Semi-arboreal apes have relatively shorter arms than their arboreal cousins. Man, being totally adapted to life necessitating travel across open grasslands, has relatively longer legs than all the other hominoids (Figure **4.4**).

Allometry – which analyses how the shape of the body changes as its overall size alters – suggests that the common ancestor of human and ape might be a medium-sized creature using a form of locomotion called 'slow climbing'. All four limbs are used to transport the animal underneath branches – a method sometimes used by gibbons and great apes today.

Keith (1923) studied the apes and monkeys living in the jungles of the Malay Peninsula and Siam. He noticed the remarkable anatomical similarity of the gibbon's spine and trunk to those of the human, while the same parts in the semnopitheque and macaque, which outwardly looked as if they might be cousins to the gibbon, were altogether different. It was not difficult for him to see that these structural features of the gibbon's body were postural adaptations. In the gibbon's flight from tree to tree his manner of progression differs altogether from that of monkeys. It is true that before starting their flight the resting posture of gibbon and monkey is much the same; both sit in a semi-erect posture, resting on their ischial callosities. In progression the gibbon uses his long arms as the chief means of support and of propulsion; he leaps with his arms, and the lower limbs are deftly used as accessory means of support or as the chief means when running along horizontal branches. The body is held, in all movements, upright to the plane of progression. The gibbon is orthograde in its gait, whereas his neighbours, the monkeys, are pronograde. As monkeys pass from branch to branch, or from tree to tree, their bodies are held parallel to the plane of motion.

Keith postulated that if a pronograde monkey were to assume the ortho-grade posture of a gibbon, the visceral contents of the abdomen would come to rest on the guardian muscles of the pelvic outlet – the levatores ani. The muscles would then contract and close the pelvic outlet by depressing the root of the tail; so long as the animal maintained the orthograde posture the muscles would have to keep contracted and the tail depressed and immobile. The pubocaudal and iliocaudal muscles have thus become postural in function when an upright position is assumed, and the depressed tail has become, except for its basal part, a useless structure. Nature would therefore get rid of it. We are certain, at least, that in the early stage of the evolution of the orthograde posture the external tail disappeared; the basal vertebrae became vestigial or coccygealized. The coccyx of the gibbon is more reduced than even that of man; it has reached its most atrophic form in the orang-utan.

If a biped loses its tail it must shorten the forward part of its body to maintain balance about the fulcrum above its hindlimbs. This has resulted in the short, thick trunks of orthograde apes compared to the long, slender trunks of pronograde monkeys, who gain their forward impetus in leaping from their hindlimbs. In the act of springing the thoracic part of their bodies is raised by extension of the loins; the lumbar part of their spine serves as a flexible lever for moving the upper part of their body on the fixed pelvic base. In the orthograde gibbon the lumbar region serves quite a different purpose. As the arms are the main organs of progression the lumbar part of the spine serves chiefly as a flexible lever for attaching the pelvis and lower limbs to the body. In the gibbon's forward flight, branches are seized by the feet for support and thus the weight of the body does come to rest temporarily on its lower limbs. Its lumbar spine serves alternately as a suspending and a supporting lever. The change from the pronograde to the orthograde posture was attended by a shortening of the lumbar region, brought about by the sacralization of the 26th body segment. In pronograde monkeys of the Old World the lumbar part forms 40–45 per cent of the presacral spine; in small orthograde apes the lumbar region varies from 30–34 per cent of the spine. With the evolution of the great anthropoid type the lumbar region of the spine became still shorter and stronger. In the chimpanzee the lumbar part forms 27 per cent of the presacral spine; in the orang-utan only 24 per cent. Man has a lumbar region measuring 32 per cent of the total length of the spine, and this represents less of a trend towards a short lumbar spine than is seen in the other anthropoids. This also applies,

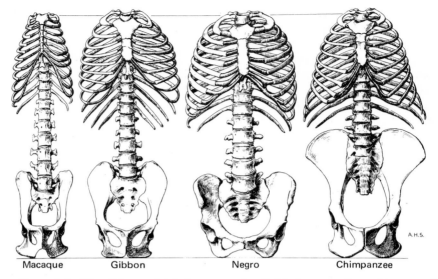

Macaque   Gibbon   Negro   Chimpanzee

Figure 4.5   The gibbon pelvis is the connecting link between anthropoid apes and quadrupedal monkeys (from Schultz, 1950)

though to a lesser extent, to the lumbar spine of the gorilla which is 29% of the total spinal length.

Le Gros Clark (1955) states that the pelvis of the large anthropoid apes contrasts with that of the monkeys in the relatively great expansion of the ilium. This is due to three trends: (1) increase in body size; (2) more powerful gluteal muscles for hip joint movements; and (3) the need for stronger abdominal muscles for visceral support. The gibbon pelvis is the connecting link between anthropoid apes and quadrupedal monkeys (Figure **4.5**).

The Cenozoic era, or the Age of Mammals, has lasted about 70 million years but man has only diverged from the gorilla and chimpanzee in the last quarter of this era. Biochemical evidence, mainly blood proteins, confirms the close affinity between man and the African apes and indicates remarkably little divergence between these species. The molecular clock suggests divergence only 5 or 6 million years ago. Almost all physical anthropologists would agree that man had diverged by 5 million years ago but some palaeontologists claim that the human line diverged much earlier. Before doubt was cast on the classification of the Miocene/Pliocene *Ramapithecus* as a hominid fossil, the date of divergence had been pushed back beyond 15 million years. Martin (1977) believes we have another situation where the resolving power of available techniques and material (semi-subjective assessment of isolated teeth and jaw fragments) leaves room for a considerable degree of personal opinion. Nevertheless he views the presently available evidence as indicating divergence between 5 and 15 million years ago.

Simons (1977) believes it is possible to clearly discern an evolutionary pathway traversing the past 14 million years from generalized hominoids to the hominids and from the hominids to the genus *Homo*. The pathway begins in Miocene times with an Old World population of apes whose fossil species was named *Dryopithecus,* a combination of the Greek for 'oak' and 'ape' reflecting the (probably correct) belief that these primates lived in the forest. Dryopithecine apes flourished over a period of some 20 million years and have been found in Europe, Asia and Africa. The fossil African apes were assigned to the genus *Proconsul,* an African member of the cosmopolitan genus *Dryopithecus.* The dryopithecines were rather generalized primates, not particularly adapted to a life of brachiation, and their posture when walking must have been essentially quadrupedal.

Fossils found in Europe and Asia since 1970 suggest that between 10 and 15 million years ago *Dryopithecus* gave rise to at least three other genera. Two of them, *Sivapithecus* and *Gigantopithecus,* were primates with a face as large as that of a modern chimpanzee or gorilla. The third genus, *Ramapithecus,* had a small face and shows the greatest similarity to later hominids. Two dozen ramapithecine jaws and teeth have been described suggesting that *Ramapithecus* had adapted to a way of life quite different from that followed by most of its forest-dwelling relatives of the dryopithecine group. Where its jaws and teeth reflect that adaptation they resemble those of the African hominid *Australopithecus.* Between the two, however, is a large gap in time. Ramapithecine species are not known to have flourished in Eurasia more recently than 8 million years ago. The earliest fossils of *Australopithecus* and *Homo* are all less than 4 million years old (Figure **4.6**).

In late Miocene times, 10 to 12 million years ago, much of Eurasia was covered with forest. The cover was not, however, tropical forest. Thus it did not provide the kind of year-long fruit production and continuous vegetative renewal that is typical of the relatively seasonless forests where apes now reside. Under these circumstances it seems likely that the larger of the Miocene apes would have found that the food available to them in the trees was inadequate, and they foraged on the ground and along the edge of the forest for small tough foods such as nuts or roots. The animal remains, associated with *Ramapithecus* at certain sites in Eurasia, suggest an even more distinct forest-fringe and wooded-savannah adaptation. Despite the gap of 4 million years *Ramapithecus* may well have had a close cousin which gave rise to the hominid genus *Australopithecus,* the 'southern ape'. These were remarkable creatures. In their limb structures they were clearly hominids but in their skulls they were rather primitive, with a small brain capacity and large jaws. They were about 1.2 m (4 feet) tall, erect and terrestrial. Their dentition was more human than ape-like, and in spite of their small brains they appear to be hominoids that have clearly evolved in the hominid rather than the pongoid direction. Many of the early members of the genus

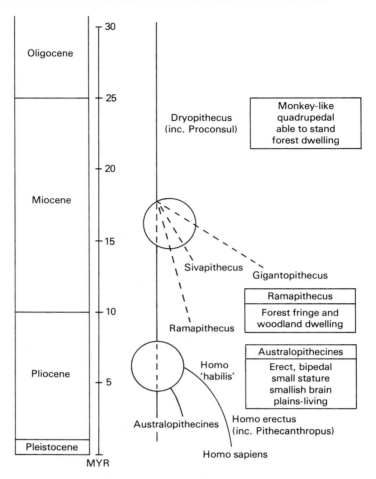

Figure 4.6   Possible evolution of *Australopithecus* and *Homo*

Homo in Africa had canine and incisor teeth somewhat larger than those typical of *Australopithecus* who was contemporary with them. The brain of the *Homo* specimens is somewhat larger, and so is their body.

Before the anthropological discoveries in East Africa over the past few years, some anthropologists had advocated a model of human evolution centring on a single, slowly evolving lineage. It now seems clear that the genus *Homo* coexisted with the genus *Australopithecus*. *Homo* may have lived in a sympatric relationship with two forms of *Australopithecus*. From crushed baboon skulls that have been found it appears likely that the australopithecines used instruments of some sort to kill the animals they hunted. Nevertheless they are probably a side-branch of human evolution that remained more or less primitive into the Pleistocene.

The explosion in the size of the human brain has been the subject of many different hypotheses, but Martin (1977) believes that the brain expanded continuously (though not necessarily uniformly) over at least 4 million years. Changes in the teeth probably occurred earlier overall. Brain expansion followed a gradual course, permitting refined integration of biological factors with emerging cultural factors over millions of years. The facial differences reflect the tripling of man's brain size. The enlarged frontal lobes have given man a more prominent forehead, and the changes in teeth have affected not only the jaw region but also other parts of the face. Selection builds powerful neck muscles in animals that fight with their canines and

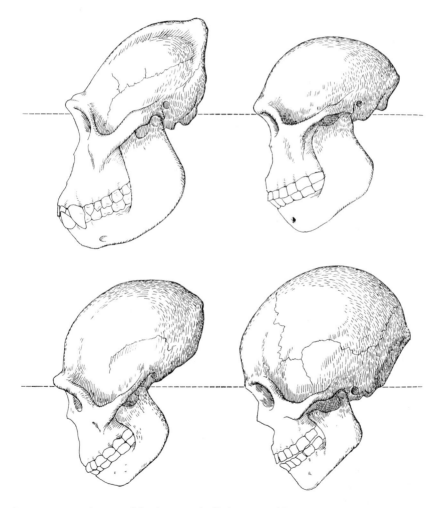

Figure 4.7   Evolution of the human skull (from Washburn, 1960)

adapts the skull to the action of these muscles. Washburn (1960) tells us that fighting is not a matter of teeth alone but also of seizing, shaking and hurling an enemy's body with the jaws, head and neck. When this behaviour is no longer necessary the jaws are shortened, there is a reduction in the ridges of bone over the eyes and a decrease in the shelf of bone in the neck area (Figure **4.7**).

It is only males who have large canine teeth and jaw muscles. The females have small canines and they hurry away with the young under the conditions in which males turn to fight. Evidence from living monkeys and apes suggests that the male's large canines are of the greatest importance to the survival of the group, and that they are particularly important in ground-living forms that may not be able to climb to safety in the trees. The early man-apes lived in open plains country and yet none of them had large canine teeth. Washburn believes that the protection of the group must have shifted from teeth to tools early in the evolution of man-apes. The skull of a man-ape is that of an ape that has lost the structure for effective fighting with its teeth. Moreover, the man-ape has transferred to its hands the functions of seizing and pulling and this has been attended by reduction of its incisors. In the man-apes the molars were very large, larger than in either ape or man. They were heavily worn, possibly because food dug from the ground with the aid of tools was very abrasive. With the men of the Middle Pleistocene, molars of human size appear along with complicated tools, hunting and fire. Pickford (1977) rejects Washburn's hypothesis that the invention of tools and weapons substituted for sharp teeth. He believes we still have to answer the question of why facial shortening should be such an important development in *Ramapithecus,* and whether it foreshadowed and eventually resulted in, the very short faces of modern humans.

The third great difference between man and the great apes is his skeletal/muscular adaptations for striding, bipedal walking. A trend towards an occasional assumption of the vertical position is documented even among some of the oldest and most primitive of today's primates but it is difficult to see precisely why only one group took to bipedal habits. Other primates, notably the baboons, have taken to a ground existence, but in spite of considerable manual dexterity they have retained a four-footed posture. Perhaps the answer can be provided by the patas monkey today which spends all of its life in open grassland. At periodic intervals, and particularly when alarmed, it stands on its hindlegs to look into the distance over the top of the surrounding tall grass. The upright stance is certainly not a way of achieving speed as monkeys, galloping on all fours, can travel at twice the speed of the fastest of modern men. Washburn believes the answer lies in the capacity for covering long distances by bipedal walking. Although the arboreal chimpanzee can run faster than man, a man can walk for many miles and this is essential for efficient hunting. In addition, the use of tools may be both the cause and effect of bipedal locomotion. Limited bipedalism left the hands sufficiently free from locomotor functions so that stones or sticks could be carried and used. The advantage that these objects gave to their users led both to more bipedalism and to more efficient tool use. Although there is fairly reliable evidence of hunting extending as far as three million years, we cannot assume that the earliest hominids were hunters, or, for that matter, gatherers. The earliest, and in some ways most significant, phases of human evolution and the reasons for the emergence of some uniquely human characteristics remain mysterious.

Among the non-human primates living today the pelvis and femur are adapted for four-footed walking. When the animal attempts to assume a

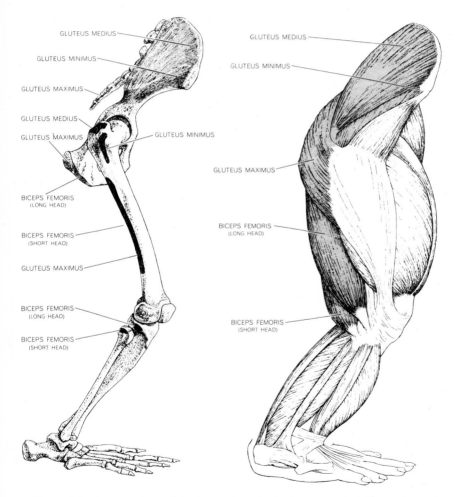

Figure 4.8   In a quadrupedal primate the principal extensors of the trunk are the gluteus medius and gluteus minimus (from Napier, 1967)

bipedal stance the trunk must be extended on the hips and as soon as the forelimbs leave the ground the body's centre of gravity has to be brought back by flexing the knees. In order to alter a bent-hip, bent-knee gait into man's erect, striding walk a number of anatomical changes must occur. These include a shortening and broadening of the pelvis, adjustments to the musculature of the hip (in order to stabilize the trunk during upright walking), a straightening of both hip and knee and considerable reshaping of the foot. The efficiency of walking is improved by an elongation of the hindlimbs with respect to the forelimbs. Napier (1967) believes the stride to be the essence of human bipedalism and the criterion by which the evolutionary status of a hominid walker must be judged. During the stance phase of the walking cycle the two muscles connecting that leg and the pelvis – the gluteus medius and gluteus minimus – contract on the stance side and brace the pelvis by cantilever action. At the same time that the pelvis is stabilized in relation to the stance leg it also rotates to the unsupported side. This rotation increases the length of the stride and, because of anatomical differences between the male and the female pelvis, for a given length of stride women must rotate the pelvis through a greater angle than do men. Rotational movement can only take place because there was a reduction in size of the iliac crests. The forward extension of the ilia provided attachments for muscles to initiate this rotation. Both the rotation and the balancing of the pelvis leave unmistakable signs on the pelvic bone and on the femur, and the distribution of weight in the foot allows the form of the foot bones to disclose the presence or absence of a striding gait.

In a quadrupedal primate the principal extensors of the trunk are the gluteus medius and gluteus minimus (Figure **4.8**). Larger primates and ones which depend for support less on their forelimbs have bulky muscles and the area of their origin – the iliac blades – increases. This accounts for the enormous extension of the iliac crests seen in chimpanzees and gorillas. With an erect posture the gluteus medius and gluteus minimus change from extensors to abductors of the trunk and the broad ilium extends forwards. The extensor function has been taken over by the gluteus maximus (Figure **4.9**). This muscle gives power to the hip joint in running, walking up a steep slope or climbing stairs and it corrects any tendency for the trunk to jack-knife on the legs. As this thigh muscle is powerfully developed in man but weakly developed in monkeys and apes, Washburn (1960) expressed the view that the modification in the form and function of the gluteus maximus initiated the change from four-footed to two-footed posture. On the other hand Napier believes the enlargement and present function of this muscle are ultimate refinements of human walking rather than initial adaptation.

The hominid stock are derived from generalized monkey-like, arboreal quadrupeds that had not become outright brachiators. *Proconsul* was quadrupedal although it occasionally raised itself on its hinder extremities. The calcaneum of *Proconsul* exhibits a remarkably well-developed basal

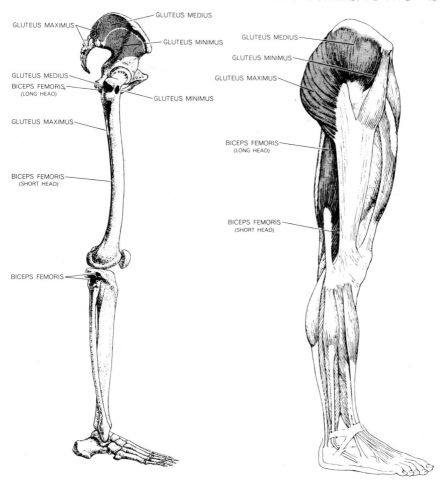

Figure 4.9 With an erect posture the extensor function is taken over by the gluteus maximus. The gluteus medius and gluteus minimus change from extensors to abductors (from Napier, 1967)

tubercle although it lies more posterior than it does in Old World monkeys and anthropoid apes. This, together with the backward extension of its main talar facet, suggests that when *Proconsul* occasionally raised itself on its hinder extremities like the modern Pongoidae it was able to throw its weight back more towards the heel and thus to balance itself in the erect posture more effectively. The conformation of the talus and calcaneum suggests that the tarsal pattern of the human foot might have been more readily derived from that of *Proconsul* than from that characteristic of any of the modern large anthropoid apes. This applies to the limb skeleton of *Pro-*

consul as a whole and it indicates strongly that the line of evolution leading directly to man did not include a distinct brachiating phase.

The australopithecines were true bipeds although their kind of upright walking should not necessarily be equated with man's heel-and-toe striding gait. The australopithecine pelvis bears positive testimony to an erect, bipedal posture. The hipbone is hominid in its overall morphology (Figure **4.10**). This is particularly true of its upper, iliac portion. The ilium is not only relatively broad but also relatively short, so that the sacral surface and acetabulum lie much nearer to each other than they do in monkeys and Pongoidae. In fact their disposition closely approximates that seen in modern man. Thus the lower part of the australopithecine ilium has undergone a shortening beyond what must have been the generalized hominoid condition. This shortening, by bringing acetabulum and sacral surface together, is an important feature in stabilization of the pelvis in the erect, bipedal posture. However, the sacral surface is comparatively much smaller that it is in man, being quite like those of the Pongoidae in its relative size. There is a marked greater sciatic notch and a prominent ischial spine. The anterior inferior iliac spine is well developed and this structure is supposed to be peculiarly related to the bipedal posture in man – particularly because of its association with the iliofemoral ligament, which prevents femoral overextension in the erect posture. Thus the upper iliac portion of the hip bone is largely hominid in morphology and indicative of adaptation to an erect, bipedal posture. On the other hand, the lower portion of the hip bone, more specifically the ischium, is much less hominid. Indeed, if anything it is

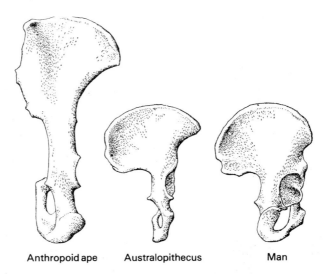

Anthropoid ape   Australopithecus   Man

Figure 4.10 The hip bone of *Australopithecus* is hominid in its overall morphology. This is particularly true of its upper, iliac portion (from Washburn, 1960)

basically simian, more closely resembling those of the anthropoid apes. Thus, the ischium is relatively long, so that ischial tuberosity and acetabulum are comparatively further apart than they are in man. Moreover, the posterior angle between ilium and ischium is longer than it is in man – another simian characteristic. Although these animals were capable of bipedal walking and running, they did not exhibit prolonged bipedal standing. Striding involves extension of the leg to a position behind the vertical axis of the spinal column. The degree of extension needed can only be achieved if the ischium of the pelvis is short. But the ischium of *Australopithecus* is long, almost as long as the ischium of an ape. Whereas in man the gluteus medius and the gluteus minimus are prime movers in stabilizing the pelvis during each stride; in *Australopithecus* this stabilizing mechanism is imperfectly evolved. The combination of both deficiencies almost entirely precludes the possibility that these hominids possessed a striding gait. For *Australopithecus* walking was something of a jog-trot. These hominids must have covered the ground with quick, rather short steps, with their knees and hips slightly bent, but as this is physiologically inefficient *Australopithecus* probably found long-distance bipedal travel impossible.

From hominid fossils discovered in Africa, McHenry and Corruccini (1976) have followed the evolution of human bipedalism. They have studied fossils of *Australopithecus* (between 1.5 and 3.0 million years old) and *Homo* (between 1.6 and 3.0 million years old). Their comparative sample consists of the femurs from 57 *Homo sapiens*, 58 chimpanzees, 66 gorillas and 34 orang-utans. As far as femoral neck length and the distance that the greater trochanter projects above the neck are concerned, all of the hominids are separate from the rest of the primates. The neck is very long in all of the fossil femora and moderately long in modern *Homo*. The human greater trochanter is lower than in the older hominoids, but in all of the early hominids the greater trochanter barely projects at all. Presumably the differences in the projection of the greater trochanter reflect differences in the function of the gluteus medius, gluteus minimus and piriformis muscles which attach on the greater trochanter. The length of the femoral neck is another feature which is associated with the abductor mechanism of the bipedal hominid hip, since the length of the neck is related to the length of the abductor lever arm. The very long femoral neck of the early hominids may imply that they had mechanically efficient lateral support mechanisms in their hips.

In the three hominid fossils classified as *Australopithecus* the femoral head diameters are uniquely small, but in the two classified as *Homo* they are more similar to extant hominids. These results can be related to what is known of australopithecine hip joint mechanics. Although the fossil hominids were bipedal, their pelvic girdles are morphologically different from modern humans in having laterally splayed iliac blades, small acetabulae and long femoral necks. Lovejoy, Heiple, and Burstein (1973) give an explanation of these differences suggesting that the evolutionary changes between the hip of the australopithecines and *Homo sapiens* is a result of encephalization; the increase in cranial size in human evolution meant a concomitant increase in size of the birth canal. The intermediate position of the two femora classified as *Homo* could be related to the intermediate cranial capacity apparent in that population. The distinctively long femoral neck of all of the early hominids indicates that the abductor lever arm was probably long which would yield a favourable biomechanical arrangement for the lateral support system in the hip which is necessary for human walking. The differences between the fossils classified as *Homo* and *Australopithecus* may imply that the hip-joint mechanics were different. A major morphological difference is the size of the femoral head. The large femoral heads might be a result of a widened birth canal. Early *Homo* has femora indistinguishable from modern man and there is good reason to assume that he attained a fully erect, bipedal posture and ran, walked and probably stood as we do today.

Thus it is a common fallacy to consider man as the only upright mammal. All existing major groups of primates include species that sit or sleep with the trunk held upright. Indeed a tendency towards an erect trunk is a basic primate characteristic. Davis (1968) believes man's outstanding postural habit is not an upright trunk but his capacity to stand for long periods with extended knees. The hominoid posture and locomotor habit were established some 12 million years ago and erect standing and walking were well established more than a million years ago. Davies believes that the popular idea that certain ailments, particularly of the trunk, arise from adoption of an erect posture may thus be incorrect. If bipedalism has been evolving and becoming more efficient over such a long period, it is difficult to imagine circumstances in which many of the pathological defects attributed to the evolution of an upright posture could have persisted in the gene pool from which the modern human population has emerged. If they were defects caused by the adoption of uprightness alone, sufficient time appears to have elapsed for them to have been selected out of the gene pool almost completely. It can only be inferred that their common appearance now is due either to the introduction of fresh genes into the pool or to some recent environmental change to which *Homo sapiens* has yet to adapt properly. Advances in functional anatomy and palaeontological thought suggest that this second alternative is probably correct.

IN SUMMARY

20. Primitive primates were tree-shrew-like animals and four-footed locomotion is still the rule for today's primates. Arboreal life needed both the ability to judge distances by sight and prehensile hands.

21. As primates evolved from animals that ran along branches to animals

that grasped branches, their trunks became relatively shorter and their limbs relatively longer.

22. Those that became outright brachiators developed long forelimbs and those that became bipedal striders developed long hindlimbs.

23. Pronograde monkeys remained a further group of quadrupeds which use flexion/extension of their spine during locomotion as they spring from branch to branch with a whip-like action of their lower spine.

24. Orthograde apes, although often similar in outward appearance to pronograde monkeys, move by using their limbs rather than their axial skeleton and not only is their trunk relatively short but they have also undergone a shortening of the length of the lumbar spine relative to pronograde monkeys.

25. Man's ancestors were non-specialized arboreal primates that became semi-arboreal and later terrestrial. They evolved from quadrupeds, to occasional bipeds, to habitual bipeds. As they became upright they became tailless, perhaps due to a need for the levatores ani to alter their action to that of supporting the abdominal contents.

26. The transition from quadrupedalism to bipedalism was accompanied

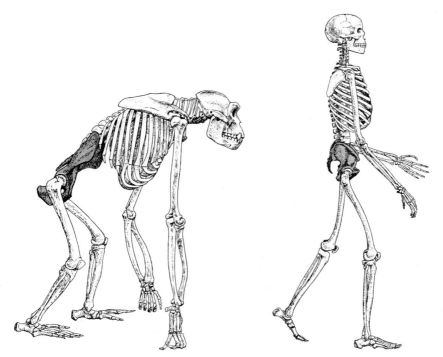

Figure 4.11 Comparison of gorilla's and man's hip bone related to difference in posture (from Napier, 1967)

by a shortening of the upper half of the hip bone with the acetabulum approaching the sacrum. The iliac crests, from which the gluteus medius and gluteus minimus are derived, shortened because these muscles no longer had to counterbalance the centre of gravity of the trunk which was well forward in semi-erect ancestors (Figure **4.11**).

27.   The transitional stage (represented by *Australopithecus*) was bipedal but probably moved with an upright jog. It had a long femoral neck, small femoral head and laterally splayed iliac blades.

28.   The spinal changes in modern man have allowed the centre of gravity of the trunk to be brought back to lie above the acetabulae. This has resulted in a lengthening of the lumbar spine and a lumbar lordosis which is peculiarly human and only associated with the final few degrees of uprightness of the trunk (Figure **4.12**).

29.   The evolution of the striding gait was accompanied by the shortening of the lower half of the hip bone. The lower limb lengthened, the femoral head increased in size and the acetabulum deepened.

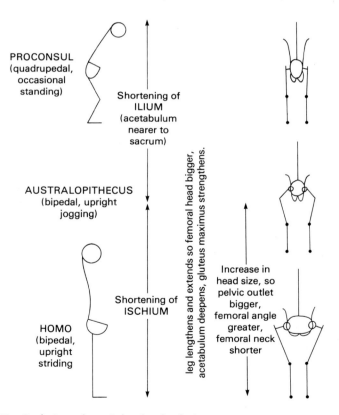

Figure 4.12   Evolution of man's lumbar lordosis

30. There was a concurrent increase in the cranial capacity and this affected the birth canal, in turn increasing the femoral angle and shortening the femoral neck.
31. In addition to shortening, the iliac crests have rotated forwards. The iliac changes together with the lengthening of the lower spine have provided the means for the trunk to be rotated in man during locomotion.
32. The form of the foot bones also disclose the degree of uprightness of the animal and the presence or absence of a striding gait.
33. The knee and hip joints also straightened and these changes together with those in the lumbar spine ensured that the later hominids could stand upright with very little muscular expenditure.

5 The uniqueness of man

If an animal is to evolve from a quadruped to a biped its centre of gravity must be moved backwards to rest above the hindlimbs. Animals of this type tend to have large tails like kangaroos and most species of birds. The centre of gravity of a kangaroo lies behind its hindlimbs and its weight is supported partly by the tail. In birds the trunk is set at an angle on the lower limbs so that the head is well in front and the tail projects backwards and balances the forward part of the trunk. The penguin's posture appears exceptional, but Joseph (1960) has observed it in detail. Although the trunk of the penguin appears to be vertical a considerable part of its lower end projects below and behind the articulation of the femur with the pelvis. In addition the penguin's lower limbs are flexed at the hips and knees (Figure **5.1**).

A bird is a balanced cantilever, the latter being constituted by the pelvic bones, drawn out and firmly welded to a long line of vertebral column. The centre of gravity is kept in a line passing through the acetabulum, and the long toes, directed fore and aft, help to preserve an unstable but well-adjusted equilibrium. The head and neck are kept small and light and their purchase on the fulcrum is under constant modification and control. A stork or heron is continually balancing itself; as the beak is thrust forward a leg stretches back. As the bird walks along its whole body sways in keeping. Thus kangaroos, birds and bipedal reptiles are able to adopt a bipedal habit by balancing the trunk over the hindlimbs. This configuration is stable at rest but unstable during locomotion. The upper body and forelimbs on the one side and the tail on the other have to engage in complicated counter-balancing to maintain equilibrium as the animal moves. If there is no tail, and hence no projection behind the fulcrum, the forward part of the body must lie directly above the fulcrum. Thus in man the trunk is approximately vertically above the lower limbs. Many four-footed animals can stand on

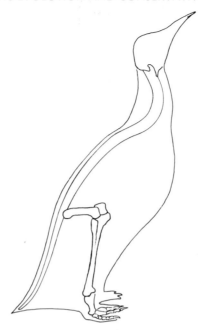

Figure 5.1 Although apparently upright and bipedal, the penguin exhibits marked flexion at the hips and knees

their hindlimbs but do not habitually do so. When they do, the segments of the hindlimbs remain partially flexed in relation to one another, for example, horses and dogs. Bears naturally adopt an upright posture not infrequently but again there is not the straightening of the segments of the limb as is seen in the normal posture of man. Other anthropoids squat when at rest, and although capable of standing on their hindlimbs only do so with flexed knees, hips and trunk.

One can readily see the way in which man's posture is unique as compared with other animals which are habitually or occasionally bipedal, but Joseph (1960) emphasized the features. In the upright position the knees and hips are extended and the vertebral column is extended above and below in the cervical and lumbar regions. This results in a general straightening of the lower limbs and body so that the segments of the body are approximately in a vertical plane. The base on which the man stands is represented by the two plantigrade feet and the centre of gravity falls within this base. By flexing the knees, hips and trunk, an approximation to the primate posture can be produced and so long as the centre of gravity falls within the base formed by the feet the body remains in equilibrium. It can be seen that the extensor muscles of the knee, hip and trunk must play an important part in producing the upright position of man.

Yamada (1962) studied bipedal rats and mice by amputating the forelegs and the tails between the third and seventh postnatal days. The animals gradually acquired the ability to stand and to walk erect but they usually assumed a half-sitting posture. Experimental bipedal animals were, in general, about 25 per cent lighter in weight than controls and the long bones of the legs were shorter and thicker than those of the controls. Radiological examination of the spine showed a tendency to a gradual increase in the degree of cervical lordosis and thoracic kyphosis with decreased lumbar kyphosis. Some even developed lumbar lordosis.

During man's evolution the transition from the quadrupedal to the bipedal state led first to the straightening and then to the inversion of the lumbar curvature which was initially concave anteriorly. The erection of the trunk has been obtained partly by backward tilting of the pelvis and partly by the bending of the lumbar column. During the development of the individual the same changes can be observed in the lumbar region (Figure 5.2). On the first day of life (a) the lumbar column is concave anteriorly. At 5 months (b) the lumbar curve is still slightly concave anteriorly but the concavity disappears at 13 months (c). From 3 years onwards the lumbar lordosis begins to appear (d), becoming obvious by 8 years (e), and assuming the definitive adult state at 10 years (f).

We have only to watch an infant trying to support its body erect when learning to walk to see reproduced the orthograde posture of a great anthropoid ape. The lower limbs are seen to be imperfectly extended, the body

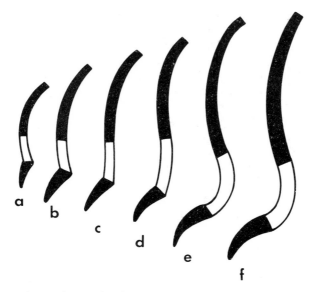

Figure 5.2 Shape of man's lumbar spine at different ages. (a) first day of life; (b) 5 months; (c) 13 months; (d) 3 years; (e) 8 years; (f) 10 years (from Kapandji, 1974)

plainly inclines forwards, and the arms stretch out to clutch at neighbouring objects for support. It is only in the second year of life that growth changes in the lumbar vertebrae make further extension of the body a permanent possibility. In addition to the appearance of the lumbar curve the loins become elongated. At birth the lumbar region measures 27 per cent of the presacral spine – the same proportion as in the chimpanzee. Elongation takes place rapidly as a child learns to walk; in the average adult the lumbar region comes to form about 32 per cent of the total length of the spine. Keith (1923) regarded the spine of a human baby, as regards the proportions of its parts and its curvatures, as in an anthropoid phase of evolution. He believed that easy and graceful carriage of the human body requires long loins to form a flexible lever on which the whole weight of the upper part of the body is poised.

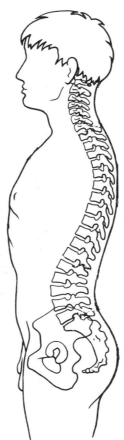

Figure 5.3   Cervical; thoracic; lumbar and sacral curves of the human spine (from Kapandji, 1974)

Schultz (1950) writes of three aspects of the general phylogenetic trend in man to bipedalism: (1) a forward shift of the spine towards the centre of the chest; (2) a backward shift of the shoulders; and (3) a bending of the spine at its junction with the hip bones. These preparations for the upright posture brought the centre of gravity of the trunk further back to lie more nearly above the acetabulae.

As well as the lumbar lordosis there are cervical, thoracic and sacral curvatures (Figure **5.3**). Kapandji (1974) believes the curvatures of the vertebral column increase its resistance to axial compression forces and because of its lumbar, thoracic and cervical curvatures it has a resistance ten times that of a straight column. He supports his theory by quoting the engineering property of curved columns as having a resistance directly proportional to the square of the number of curvatures plus one.

On the other hand, Steindler (1955) looked upon the S-shaped human spine as a spring, damping vertical impacts by increasing all its curves. Asmussen and Klausen (1962) rejected this teleological view and emphasized that the thoracic kyphosis is a feature common to all mammals, whereas the lumbar lordosis is especially human and is connected with the erect posture on straight legs. They showed that the angle representing the kyphosis increases slightly with age, whereas the angle representing the lordosis apparently first increases but then, from age 15 years, seems to decrease. The trend seemed to go in the direction of a flatter low back with a more pronounced kyphosis in adults as compared with children.

On balance it seems probable that the lordosis is an adaptation to upright

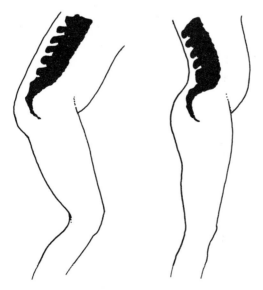

Figure 5.4   The lordosis is an adaptation to upright stance with straight knees

stance with straight knees (Figure **5.4**). As a lumbar lordosis is neither seen in apes nor in man with a forward tilt and bent knees, we conclude it has been produced by the final few degrees of straightness. Being a mammal, man is endowed with a thoracic kyphosis surrounding his respiratory cage. To bring the centre of gravity of the trunk above the hips, the lumbar spine must bend backwards upon itself. The centres of gavity of the various ascending portions of the body must align themselves vertically above the hips to allow for prolonged standing. The lumbar lordosis, therefore, is more pronounced in conditions such as abdominal obesity and pregnancy which would otherwise cause the abdominal centre of gravity to be placed further forward. In pregnancy the shift of the centre of gravity is offset by leaning backwards.

The cervical lordosis likewise brings the centre of gravity of the head posteriorly. The head is in equilibrium when the eyes look horizontally and in this position the plane of the bite is also horizontal. Nevertheless the centre of gravity lies in front of the fulcrum (the occipital condyles) when the head is in equilibrium and the posterior neck muscles must constantly counterbalance the weight of the head as it tends to tilt forwards.

De Seze (1974) showed the features of the lumbar lordosis and the vertebral column at rest (Figure **5.5**).

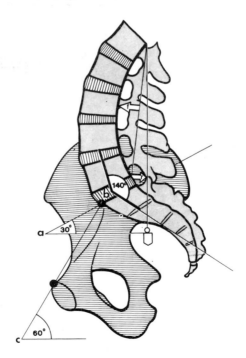

Figure 5.5 The features of lumbar lordosis and of the vertebral column at rest (see text for key) (from Kapandji, 1974)

(1) The angle of the sacrum (a), formed between the horizontal and the plane containing the superior aspect of S_1, averages 30°;

(2) The lumbosacral angle (b), lying between the axis of L_5 and the sacral axis, averages 140°;

(3) The angle of pelvic tilt (c), formed by the horizontal and the line joining the promontory to the superior border of the pubic symphysis, averages 60°;

(4) The index of lumbar lordosis (white arrow f) can be determined by joining the superoposterior border of L_1 to the posteroinferior border of L_5. The perpendicular to this line is usually maximal at L_3 and represents the index of lordosis. It is greater as lordosis is more marked and almost disappears when the column is straight. It can rarely become inverted.

(5) The posterior projection (white arrow r) represents the distance between the posteroinferior border of L_5 and the vertical line passing through the superoposterior border of L_1. It can be positive if the lumbar column is thrown backwards; or negative if the column if flexed.

Kapandji (1974) quoted Delmas when he showed the functional signific-ance of certain vertebrae in maintaining the erect position (Figure **5.6**). L_3 is pulled posteriorly by muscles arising from the sacrum and ilium and can serve as origin for the thoracic muscles. Therefore L_3 is important in the mechanics of the vertebral column at rest, the more so as it coincides with the apex of the lumbar curvature and its superior and inferior surfaces are parallel and horizontal. It is the lowest truly mobile lumbar vertebra as L_4 and L_5, strongly bound to the ilium and sacrum, represent more a static than a dynamic bridge between sacrum and vertebral column. The twelfth thoracic vertebra, on the other hand, is the point of inflexion between the lumbar and thoracic curvatures. It acts as a swivel and its body is more massive than its vertebral arch, covered posteriorly by the vertebral muscles as they course along without inserting. Delmas considered T_{12} as the swivel of the vertebral axis.

Delmas also classified vertebral columns into those with pronounced curvatures (dynamic types) and those with attenuated curvatures (static types). He described a correlation between the type of column and the structure of the sacrum and its articular facet. When the curvatures of the vertebral column are pronounced the sacrum lies horizontally and its articular facet is markedly buckled on itself and deep. The sacroiliac joint is highly mobile resembling the typical synovial joints and he believed it represents overadaptation to the biped state. When the curvatures of the vertebral column are poorly developed the sacrum is almost vertical and its articular facet is enlongated vertically, slightly buckled on itself and almost flat. This structural constitution corresponds to a joint of low mobility, like the secondary cartilaginous joints. It is often seen in children and closely resembles that found in the primates. During evolution from primates to

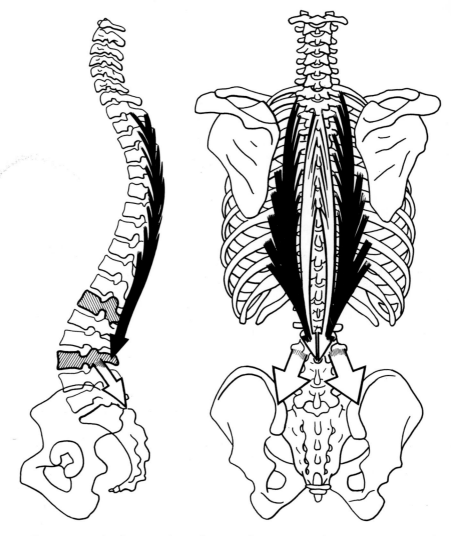

Figure 5.6   The functional significance of certain vertebrae in maintaining the erect position (from Kapandji, 1974)

man the caudal segment of the articular facet becomes longer and assumes greater significance than the cranial segment. In man the angle between these two segments can attain 90°, while in primates the articular facet is only minimally buckled (Figure **5.7**).

In the centre of the articular surface of the sacrum there is a curved furrow bordered by two long crests and corresponding to an arc of a circle whose centre lies on the transverse tubercle of S_1 (black cross in Figure **5.8**). This

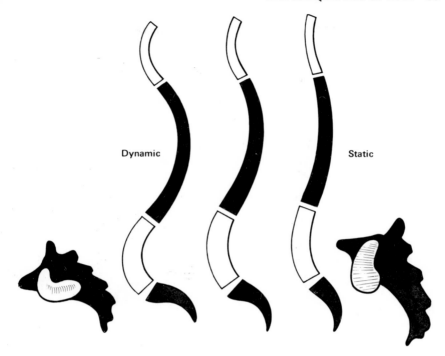

Figure 5.7 Variation of angle between two segments of sacral articular facet (from Kapandji, 1974)

tubercle is the point of insertion of some powerful ligaments of the sacroiliac joint. The articular surface of the ilium corresponds to the articular surface of the sacrum. It lies on the posterosuperior part of the medial aspect of the iliac bone, just posterior to the iliopectineal line, which in turn forms part of the pelvic brim. It is crescent-shaped, concave posterosuperiorly, and is lined by cartilage. Its long axis contains a long crest lying between two furrows. This curved crest corresponds to an arc of a circle whose centre lies approximately at the sacral tuberosity (black cross). This tuberosity is the point of insertion of the powerful sacroiliac ligaments.

Mednick (1955) studied the internal architecture of chimpanzee and human pelves. In terms of thick–thin bone areas the chimpanzee has a thick column from the posterior superior spine to the ischial tuberosity; the iliac alae are thinner. In man there is thick bone from the sacroiliac articulation to the acetabulum; the external table of bone from the iliac tubercle to the acetabulum is even thicker (Figure **5.9**).

In the chimpanzee the split-line pattern shows the inner and the outer patterns to be the same (Figure **5.10**). In man the inner pattern is as in the chimpanzee but the outer pattern is different; in the chimpanzee there are two radiations, one from the sacroiliac articulation to the ischial tuberosity,

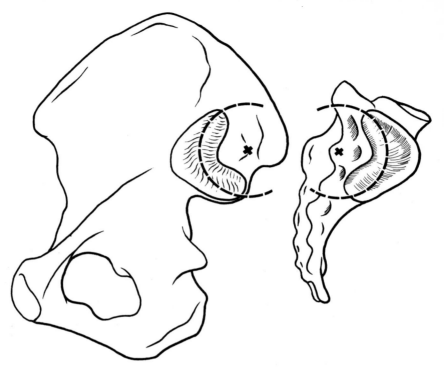

Figure 5.8   The articular surface of the sacroiliac joint (see text for key) (from Kapandji, 1974)

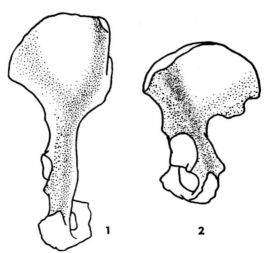

Figure 5.9   Areas of thick-thin bone in pelvis of chimpanzee (1) and human (2). Stippling shows thicker bone (from Mednick, 1955)

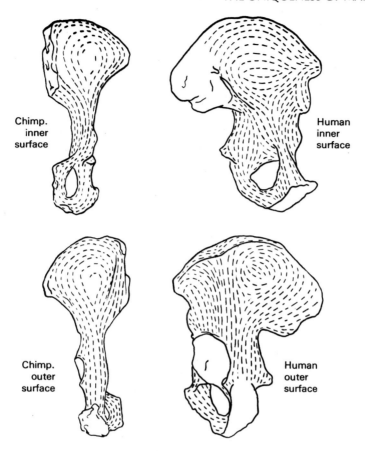

Chimp.
inner
surface

Human
inner
surface

Chimp.
outer
surface

Human
outer
surface

Figure 5.10 Split-line patterns in the pelvic bone (from Mednick, 1955)

the other from the upper border of the acetabulum to the iliac crest. In man there are three radiations: the first from the anterior superior iliac spine to the upper acetabulum, the second from the sacroiliac articulation to the ischial tuberosity, the third from below the iliac tuberosity to the posterior margin of the acetabulum (the third corresponds to the thick column of bone). The thicker bone columns (or pillars) and the split-line force patterns are all evidence of a shift from semi-quadrupedal to bipedal locomotion. First there was a widening, shortening and bending back of the ilium; then 'pillar development' in internal iliac structure plus changes in iliac tubercle; then changes in ramus and tuberosity of ischium, so that the hamstrings, with a higher-placed attachment, had enhanced extensor action in full extension of the hip. Thus three stages may be envisioned: (1) erect posture, due to changes in size and the proportions of the ilium; (2) balance, due to

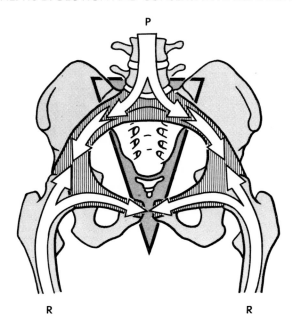

Figure 5.11   Transmission of forces from vertebral column to the lower limbs (see text for key) (from Kapandji, 1974)

iliac tubercle and iliac pillar changes; and (3) nearer perfect bipedalism due to ischial shortening and tubercle changes.

In man the bony pelvis transmits forces from the vertebral column to the lower limbs (Figure **5.11**). The weight (P) supported by L_5 is distributed equally along the alae of the sacrum and through the ischial tuberosities towards the acetabulum. Part of the reaction of the ground to the body weight (R) is transmitted to the acetabulum by the neck and head of the femur. The rest is transmitted across the horizontal ramus of the pubic bone and is counterbalanced at the symphysis pubis by a similar force from the other side. These lines of force form a complete ring along the pelvic brim. Therefore the complex system of bony trabeculae in the pelvic bones corresponds to the lines of force. As the sacrum is broader above than below it can be taken as a wedge which fits vertically between the two iliac bones. The heavier the weight it is bearing the more tightly the sacrum is held, and it is therefore a self-locking system.

IN SUMMARY

34.   Birds must keep their centres of gravity directly over the acetabulae by continually counterbalancing the foreparts and hindparts of the trunk.

35.   Non-human bipeds usually stand with flexed hips and knees. Man's knees and hips are extended and his lumbar spine, which in infancy is concave anteriorly, develops a lumbar extension to become concave posteriorly (lumbar lordosis).

36.   Other phylogenetic trends shown by man to bipedalism include a forward shift of the spine towards the centre of the chest and a backward shift of the shoulders. All these preparations for the upright posture brought the centre of gravity of the trunk further back to lie more nearly above the acetabulae.

6

The anatomy of posture

Kapandji (1974) has described the functions of the ligaments of the lower spine and its junction with the pelvis in man so well that this account is taken almost entirely from his book.

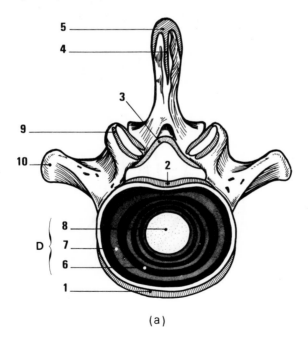

(a)

Figure 6.1a & **6.1b** Horizontal section and lateral view of spine showing ligaments. (see text for key) (from Kapandji, 1974)

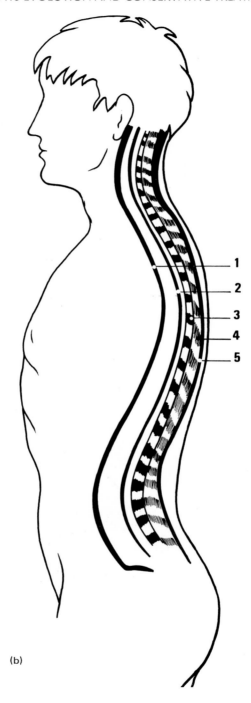

1
2
3
4
5

(b)

Between the sacrum and the base of the skull there are 24 movable vertebrae linked together by fibrous ligaments. A horizontal section and a lateral view show the following ligaments (Figure **6.1a** and **b**):

(1) the anterior longitudinal ligament, stretching from the basi-occiput to the sacrum on the anterior surfaces of the vertebrae;
(2) the posterior longitudinal ligament, extending from the basi-occiput to the sacral canal on the posterior aspect of the vertebrae.

These long ligaments are interlinked at each vertebral level by the intervertebral disc (D) which is made up of two parts, the peripheral annulus fibrosus formed by concentric layers of fibrous tissue (6 and 7) and centrally, the nucleus pulposus (8).

Other ligaments connect the arches of adjacent vertebrae:
(3) the ligamentum flavum, thick, strong and yellow;
(4) the interspinous ligament;
(5) the supraspinous ligament which is poorly defined in the lumbar region but is quite distinct in the neck;
(9) the anterior and posterior ligaments of the articular processes, strengthening the capsular ligaments;
(10) the intertransverse ligament attached to the superior surface of each transverse process.

The anterior longitudinal ligament (1, Figure **6.2a**) is inserted into the anterior aspects of both the individual vertebral bodies (2) and the intervertebral discs (3) leaving a potential space (4) where osteophytes are formed in osteoarthritis.

The posterior longitudinal ligament (5) is inserted into the posterior aspect of the intervertebral disc (6), but not into the posterior surface of the vertebra, thus leaving a free space (7) traversed by a paravertebral venous plexus. The concavity of each festoon is related to a pedicle (10, Figure **6.2b**). The sagittal section (Figure **6.2a**) shows the intervertebral disc with its annulus fibrosus (8) and its nucleus pulposus (9).

The ligamentum flavum (11 and transected 12) is inserted inferiorly into the superior border of the underlying lamina and superiorly into the medial aspect of the overlying lamina. Its medial edge fuses with the contralateral ligament in the midline and completely closes the vertebral canal. Anteriorly and laterally it covers the capsular and the anteromedial ligaments (14) of the joints between the articular processes.

The spinous processes are joined by the powerful interspinous ligament (15), continuous posteriorly with the supraspinous ligament (16) which is attached to the tips of the spinous processes. The intertransverse ligament (17) is well developed in the lumbar region (Figure **6.2c**).

Figure **6.2c** is the vertebral arch viewed from in front and the upper

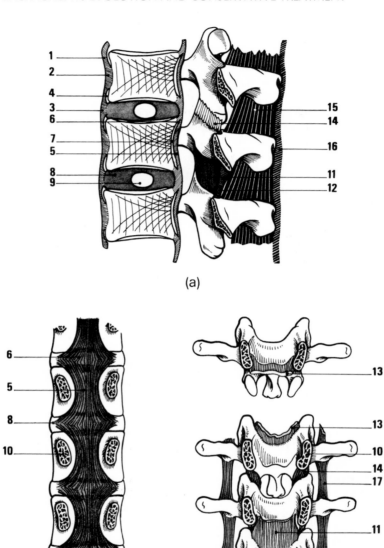

(a)

(b)

(c)

Figure 6.2a, b, c Sagittal section after removal of the laminae on the left. Frontal section taken through the pedicles. Vertebral arch viewed from in front (see text for key) (from Kapandji, 1974)

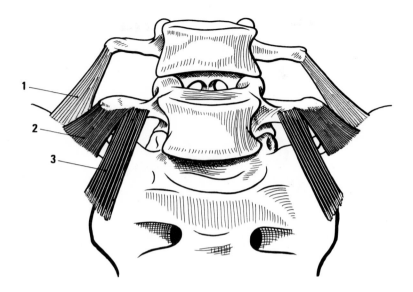

Figure 6.3   The iliolumbar ligaments seen from in front (see text for key) (from Kapandji, 1974)

vertebra has been detached after sectioning the ligamentum flavum (13). Between the second and third vertebrae the ligament has been totally removed to show the capsule and the anteromedial ligament of the joint between the articular processes (14) and the spinous process.

The last two lumbar vertebrae are joined directly to the iliac bone by the iliolumbar ligaments seen in Figure **6.3** from in front. The superior band (1) is attached to the tip of the transverse process of L_4 and runs inferiorly, laterally and posteriorly to be inserted into the iliac crest. The inferior band (2) is attached to the tip of the transverse process of L_5 and runs inferiorly and laterally to be inserted into the iliac crest. Occasionally the inferior band is divided into an iliac band (2) and a sacral band (3). The strength of the iliolumbar ligaments helps to limit movement at the sacroiliac joint by restricting lateral flexion rather than flexion and extension.

A posterior view of the pelvis (Figure **6.4**) shows the superior band (1) and the inferior band (2) of the iliolumbar ligaments and on the right side the intermediate plane of the sacroiliac ligaments. This comprises:

(3) a ligament running from the iliac crest to the transverse tubercle of S_1;

(4) the four ligaments running from the posterior aspect of the iliac crest to the sacral tubercles.

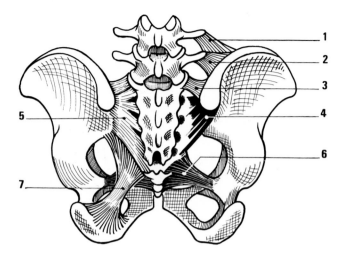

Figure 6.4 Posterior view of pelvis to show iliolumbar ligaments, intermediate the anterior planes of sacroiliac ligaments, sacrospinous ligament and sacrotuberous ligament. (see text for key) (from Kapandji, 1974)

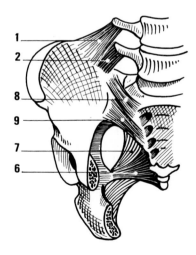

Figure 6.5 Anterior view of pelvis to show iliolumbar, sacrospinous, sacrotuberous, anterosuperior sacroiliac and anteroinferior sacroiliac ligaments (see text for key) (from Kapandji, 1974)

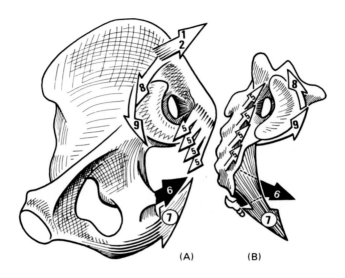

Figure 6.6   Right sacroiliac joint, opened by rotation of the constituent bones about a vertical axis, and its ligaments (see text for key) (from Kapandji, 1974)

On the left side is the anterior plane of the sacroiliac ligaments (5) consisting of a fibrous band running from the posterior edge of the iliac bone to the articular tubercles of the sacrum.

The sacrospinous ligament (6) runs obliquely from the ischial spine to the lateral border of the sacrum and coccyx. The sacrotuberous ligament (7) crosses obliquely the posterior aspect of the former ligament as it runs from the posterior border of the iliac bone and the coccyx to the ischial tuberosity and the medial tip of the ascending ramus of the ischium.

An anterior view of the pelvis (Figure **6.5**) shows the iliolumbar (1 and 2), the sacrospinous (6) and the sacrotuberous ligaments (7), and in addition the anterosuperior (8) and anteroinferior (9) sacroiliac ligaments.

The beautifully descriptive figure (Figure **6.6**) shows the right sacroiliac joint, opened by rotation of the constituent bones about a vertical axis, and its ligaments. The medial surface of the iliac bone (*A*) and the lateral surface (*B*) of the sacrum are exposed. The ligaments numbered in the previous figures are wrapped around the joint. The short axial ligament is shown attached to both the iliac bone and the sacrum immediately posterior to the sacroiliac articular surfaces.

The posterior muscles of the trunk are arranged in three planes. The deep plane consists of muscles that are short and directly attached to the vertebrae (Figure **6.7a** and **b**). These paravertebral muscles are the transversospinalis (1), the interspinalis muscles (2), the spinalis muscles (3), the

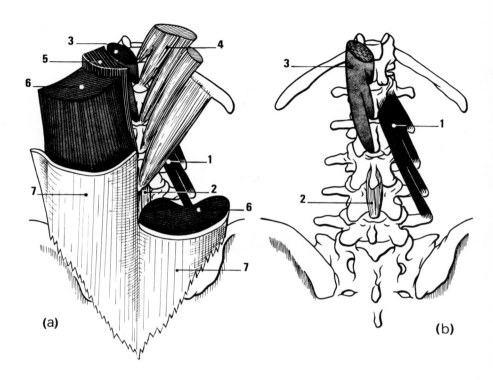

Figure 6.7a & **6.7b** The posterior muscles of the trunk (see text for key) (from Kapandji, 1974)

longissimus (5) and the iliocostalis (6). In the lower part of the trunk all the muscles form a common mass attached to a thick tendinous sheath which is continuous with the aponeurosis of the latissimus dorsi (7).

The intermediate plane is comprised of the serratus posterior inferior (4), which arises from the first three lumbar vertebrae and the last two thoracic vertebrae and is inserted into the lateral aspect of the last three or four ribs.

The superficial plane is made up of the latissimus dorsi (7), which arises from the thick lumbar aponeurosis and forms a broad sheet covering the posterolateral part of the lower thorax on its way to its humeral insertion.

The action of the posterior muscles is related to extension of the lumbar vertebral column. When the sacrum is fixed they powerfully extend the lumbar and thoracic vertebral columns at the lumbosacral joint and at the thoracolumbar joint respectively. In addition they accentuate the lumbar lordosis as they span completely or partially the two ends of the lumbar

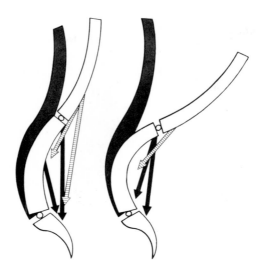

Figure 6.8   Action of the posterior trunk muscles (from Kapandji, 1974)

curvature. They pull the lumbar column posteriorly and increase its curvature (Figure **6.8**).

The lateral muscles of the trunk are the quadratus lumborum and the psoas. The quadratus lumborum viewed from in front (1, Figure **6.9a**) laterally flexes the trunk to the same side, an action which is helped by the internal oblique and external oblique abdominal muscles. The psoas (2) lies anterior to the quadratus; it arises from T_{12} and the lumbar vertebrae and runs an oblique course inferiorly and laterally to gain insertion into the tip of the lesser trochanter. If the hip joint is fixed by other muscles the psoas laterally flexes the lumbar vertebral column to the same side and rotates it contralaterally (Figure **6.9b**). Furthermore as it is attached to the summit of the lumbar curvature, it flexes the vertebral column relative to the pelvis and accentuates the lumbar lordosis (Figure **6.9c**).

The two rectus muscles lie in the anterior abdominal wall on either side of the midline (Figure **6.10**). The transversus abdominis forms the deepest layer of the lateral abdominal muscles. It is attached posteriorly to the lumbar vertebrae and as it passes forwards it crosses the midline to merge with its fellow on the opposite side. Its lowest fibres end on the public symphysis and join those of the internal oblique to form the conjoint tendon (Figure **6.11**).

The internal oblique makes up the intermediate layer of the muscles of the abdominal wall. The muscles fibres are attached to the iliac crest, to the lower ribs and to an aponeurosis along the lateral edge of the rectus. The

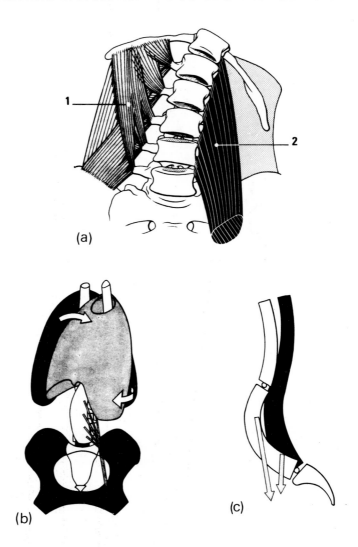

Figure 6.9a, b, c   The lateral muscles of the trunk (see text for key) (from Kapandji, 1974)

lowest fibres, attached directly to the inguinal ligament, form the conjoint tendon along with the transversus before gaining attachment to the superior border of the pubic symphysis and the pubic crest (Figure **6.12**).

The external oblique forms the superficial muscle layer of the abdominal wall arising from the lower ribs and giving rise to the aponeurosis along the lateral border of the rectus (Figure **6.13**).

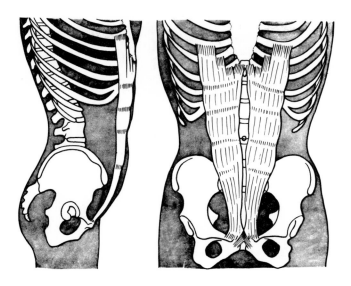

Figure 6.10   The two rectus muscles (from Kapandji, 1974)

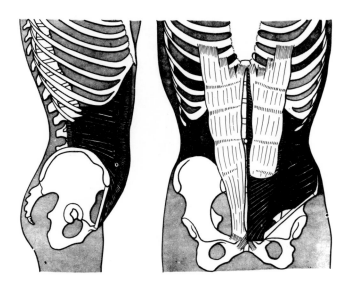

Figure 6.11   The transversus abdominis muscle (from Kapandji, 1974)

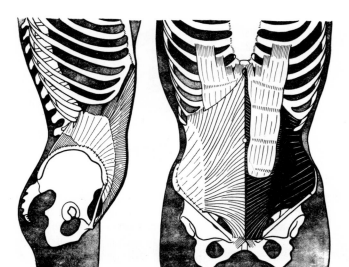

Figure 6.12   The internal oblique muscle (from Kapandji, 1974)

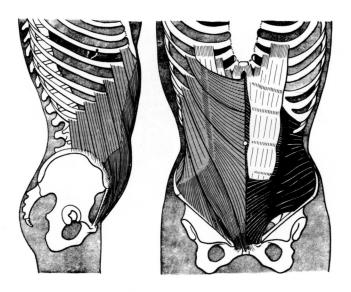

Figure 6.13   The external oblique muscle (from Kapandji, 1974)

The lateral muscles are arranged in three layers with their muscle fibres running in different directions: in the deep layer (transversus) the fibres are transverse; in the intermediate layer (internal oblique) they are oblique superiorly and medially; in the superficial layer (external oblique) they are oblique inferiorly and medially.

Joseph (1960) wrote of two schools of thought regarding the way in which stability at the joints in the standing-at-ease position is maintained. On the one hand it is thought that the action of opposing groups of muscles is the main factor and that the role of the ligaments is to prevent overstretching. As the spine is constructed from many movable parts, and even during quiet standing it is subject to postural sway, it must be kept in position by active forces which counteract the pull of gravity and the other forces acting on it. These active forces are muscular and they adapt to the changing positions of the body by contracting reflexly. The 'stays' or 'guys' are represented by the muscles of the trunk, the abdominal muscles in front and to the sides, and the erectores spinae on the back. The other school of thought places more emphasis on the relationship of the line of weight (the vertical through the centre of gravity) to the ankle, knee, hip and spinal joints. By electromyography, using skin electrodes pasted to the skin over the muscles, it is possible to detect whether or not underlying muscles are active and thereby to help solve this controversy.

In the standing-at-ease position the line of weight falls in front of the ankle joint in most of the subjects studied (Figure **6.14**). As there are no passive structures such as ligaments at the back of the ankle joint to maintain dorsiflexion, it is not surprising that electromyography shows there to be continuous activity in the soleus (and often also in the gastrocnemius) whilst standing at ease, and no activity in the tibialis anterior. Occasional bursts of

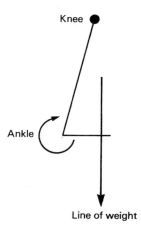

Figure 6.14   In the standing at ease position the line of weight falls in front of the ankle joint

high amplitude potentials were observed by Joseph from the muscles of some women while they were wearing high heels due to instability in their posture. The line of weight in a woman wearing high heels bore no constant relationship to her line of weight when low heels were worn but the wearing of high heels produces plantar flexion of the foot which shortens the distance between the line of action of the calf muscles and the ankle joint. Thus a more powerful contraction of the soleus is necessary to maintain the upright position.

On swaying forwards 5° the activity in soleus increased; on swaying backwards 5° the activity in that muscle decreased, and then a sudden burst of activity from tibialis anterior was seen. Throughout the range of swaying either the muscles of the front or the back of the leg were active, and there was no position when muscle activity was not necessary to maintain the upright position.

Most authors agree that the line of weight passes a little in front of the transverse axis of the knee joints and that this relationship is retained throughout normal swaying (Figure **6.15**). Thus one would expect the quadriceps femoris to be relaxed and the hamstrings contracted in the standing-at-ease position. However, in the standing position no further extension at the knee joint is possible and therefore non-contractile structures may bear the body weight on their own. Electromyographic studies confirm that in the majority of men and women, and in the latter while wearing high heels, there is no detectable activity in the quadriceps femoris or hamstrings. If the line of weight is shifted forwards the hamstrings

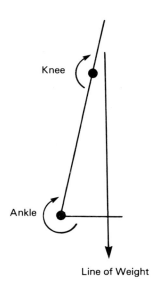

Line of Weight

Figure 6.15 The line of weight passes a little in front of the knee joints

become active, if it shifts backwards the quadriceps femoris contract to prevent flexion of the knees which would occur due to gravity. Nevertheless under normal swaying there is an absence of detectable potentials in both muscle groups as the knee is self-locking until the line of weight falls behind the joint.

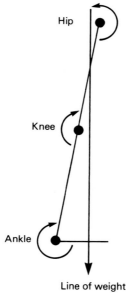

Figure 6.16   The line of weight passes 2 cm behind the axis of the hip joints

Akerblom (1948) showed that the line of weight usually passes 2 cm or so behind the axis of the hip joints (range 0 to 4 cm, mean 1.8 cm) in the ordinary standing position and the amount of further extension possible at the hip joints was small (Figure **6.16**). Thus he maintained that the body was usually balanced over the hip joints in a position of unstable equilibrium. Joseph (1960) examined the hip extensors (gluteus medius, minimus and maximus) and a hip flexor (iliopsoas) electromyographically in the standing-at-ease position. In all subjects the recordings from the extensors showed no activity but similar results were obtained from the iliopsoas except when the subjects contracted their abdominal muscles.

On the other hand other workers, including Basmajian (1958), Close (1964) and Nachemson (1966), have shown continuous electromyographic activity in the iliopsoas in both a sitting and standing upright posture (Figure **6.17**). Furthermore Snidjers (1969) developed a method of describing the form of the spine mathematically using lateral and anterioposterior radiographs. In all the spines he examined in an unconstrained erect posture he found a curvature in the lumbar area indicating a forward moment acting

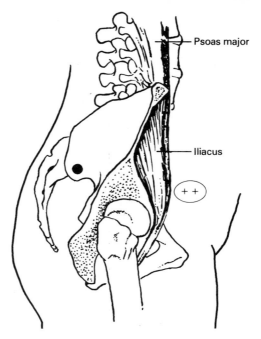

Figure 6.17 Moment of force procured by the m. ilio-psoas in natural erect posture (after Basmajian, 1961)

around the hip joint. He was convinced that this moment was produced by the iliopsoas muscle.

Joseph (1960) found that shifting the line of weight forwards initiated potentials in the hamstrings but not in the gluteal muscles. He therefore disagreed with the view that a subject standing at ease is in a state of unstable equilibrium because he did not obtain activity in the extensors or flexors of the hip during over 5 min of continuous standing. Akerblom's (1948) observations showing that the line of weight passes behind the axis of the hip joints provide a plausible explanation as to why the extensors show no activity. As the potential for further extension at the hip joint is small in the standing position, extension may well be prevented by ligaments rather than the hip flexors. These findings suggest that the hip is in equilibrium, unstable to flexion large enough to move the line of weight in front of the joint but stable to extension.

As the line of weight (represented by P in Figure **6.18**) passes only 2 cm behind the reaction of the ground (R) transmitted by the femora, the pelvis rests on the femoral heads with only small amounts of muscular activity and ligamentous tension. This is not the situation existing at the sacroiliac joints. Here the centre of gravity falls well in front of the articulation and the spine tends to rotate forwards on the pelvis (Figure **6.19**). This rotation has to be

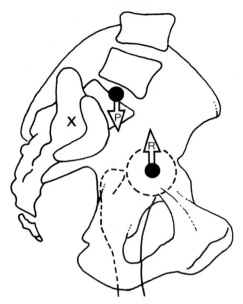

Figure 6.18   Relationship between line of weight (P), hip joint and sacroiliac joint (see text for key) (adapted from Kapandji, 1974)

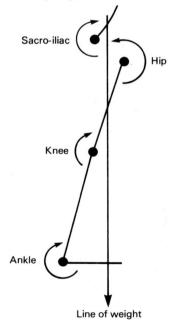

Figure 6.19   The line of weight falls well in front of the sacroiliac joint and the spine tends to rotate forwards on the pelvis

resisted by ligaments and muscles attached to both the spine and the pelvis. The ligaments preventing this rotation are the anterior sacroiliac ligaments and the sacrospinous and sacrotuberous ligaments (see Figure **6.6**). Once the sacroiliac joints have been relatively immobilized by these ligaments,

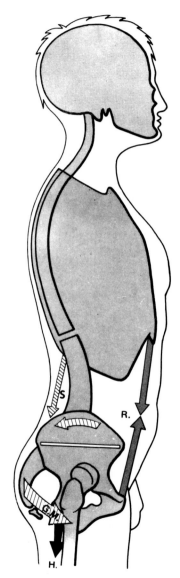

Figure 6.20 Activators of the sacroiliac joints and lumbar lordosis (see text for key) (from Kapandji, 1974)

the lower spine and pelvis move in unison. For example, forward leaning by the subject tends to rotate the whole pelvis forwards so that ligaments and muscles acting upon both the pelvis and legs (Figure **6.20**), the gluteus maximus (GM) and hamstring muscles (H), must resist the forward rotation. When the lower spine, pelvis and femora are stabilized the abdominal muscles, particularly the rectus muscles (R), are able to flex the trunk on the fixed pelvis. Extension is provided by the paravertebral muscles (S) which pull back the upper lumbar vertebrae. During standing the paravertebral muscles bring the centre of gravity of the trunk back over the hip joint to lessen the moments acting on the sacroiliac and hip joints. Thus the abdominal muscles flatten the lumbar lordosis and the paravertebral muscles increase the degree of lumbar lordosis. In addition contraction of the hamstrings and gluteus maximus rotate the pelvis backwards and help to flatten the lordosis.

The activity of the muscles of the back in the standing-at-ease position varies considerably at different levels of the trunk and depends on whether the segment above the level studied tends to fall forwards or backwards under the influence of gravity. Nevertheless one may derive a general principle from the studies of the muscles of the lower limb and state that if the line of weight of the segment above the joints which are being con-sidered passes in front of the transverse axis of these joints, the muscles of the back will be contracted, and if the opposite is the case these muscles will show an absence of detectable electrical activity. In the former case there may be a passive mechanism preventing flexion and as a result the extensor muscles would not show detectable activity. Asmussen and Klausen (1962) recorded electromyographs simultaneously from the abdominal muscles (rectus abdominis) and the lumbar portion of the erectores spinae. When standing quietly, only one set of muscles is active while the antagonists are silent electrically. In the majority of cases (75 per cent) it was the muscles of the back that counteracted gravity.

The authors deduced that the line of gravity for that part of the body above the lumbar lordosis must pass ventrally to the axis for sagittal movements in the lumbar spine. This differed from the previously accepted view that the line of gravity intersects with all four curves of the spine. The line of gravity for the upper part of the body passes very close to the outer ear opening in the erect posture. Taking this into account, the approximate position of the line of gravity for the trunk, the head and the arms can be determined by means of roentgenography or by anthropometric measurements. X-ray pictures showed that in adults the line of gravity was located 1 cm ventral to the centre of the 4th lumbar vertebral body. This confirms that gravity tends to straighten the lumbar lordosis, not, as postulated previously, to aggravate it. Correspondingly, from anthropometric measurements on 201 boys Asmussen and Heebøll-Nielsen (1959) found that the course of the line through the outer ear opening passed about 1 cm in front of the lumbar

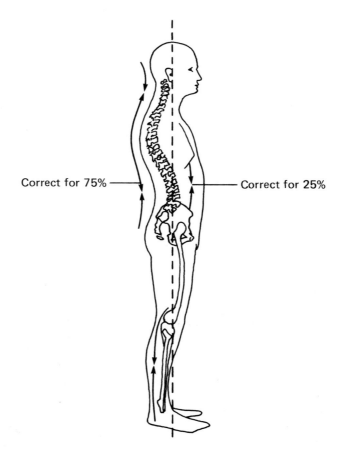

Correct for 75% ————————— ————— Correct for 25%

Figure 6.21   The line of weight in relation to the standing at ease posture and the muscles which are active in maintaining the posture.

lordosis (centre of L_4). Only where the abdominal muscles are active during quiet standing must it be expected that the line of gravity will pass dorsal to the transverse axis of movement in the lumbar spine. These cases represented 20–25 per cent of adults, a figure which corresponds entirely to the results obtained from the anthropometric measurements.

The standing-at-ease posture is shown in Figure **6.21** with the line of weight and the muscles which are active in maintaining this posture.

Lucas (1970) studied the erectores spinae muscles not only during standing at rest but also during various activities. His electromyographic recordings showed slight activity of all the muscles while the subjects were standing at rest and this activity was increased by swaying of the trunk. During flexion, all muscles tested were active and reflected their antigravity function. During rest in the fully flexed position, muscle activity decreased remarkably. When the trunk was extended to an erect position, there was an initial burst of activity which rapidly decreased as the extended position was attained. When the subject hyperextended, muscle activity virtually ceased until the subject was asked to forcibly hyperextend as much as possible. At that point there was a marked increase in activity which again nearly ceased as the subject returned to a normal standing position.

The erectores spinae muscles were generally active during ipsilateral rotation; during contralateral rotation, the rotatores and multifidus displayed a complementary relationship. During return to the normal position, there was a marked decrease in muscle activity, indicating that an automatic spring-like recoil was produced by the force resulting from the release from tension of the passive soft tissues.

During ipsilateral flexion, or side-bending, activity was observed in all of the back muscles of four subjects, indicating that the trunk is pulled over to one side as opposed to its forward flexion when the trunk is lowered in opposition to the force of gravity. In the fifth subject, who was tall and thin and the most limber of the group, the reverse was true, as the muscles behaved in an antigravity fashion. Forced lateral flexion required ipsilateral hyperactivity in the muscles of all five subjects.

During lateral bending in the flexed position, there is almost continual muscle activity. The same is true of rotation in the forward flexed position. Continual activity is no doubt due to the awkward position and the need for additional trunk stability to perform such complex manoeuvres.

In all subjects, however, lateral flexion and rotation during hyperextension required little muscle activity except for lateral bending and rotation and indicated less need for trunk stabilization while the subject was performing those acrobatics.

Similar additional studies of the abdominal muscles indicate that they, too, act in an antigravity fashion except when called upon to overcome passive resistance of soft tissues such as ligaments and visceral structures.

IN SUMMARY

37. In man's standing-at-ease posture the vertical through the body's centre of gravity passes in front of the ankle joint. Electromyographic studies confirm continuous activity in the calf muscles to maintain this stance. On swaying forwards activity in the calf muscles increases; on swaying backwards the activity in these muscles decreases and the tibialis anterior suddenly takes over.

38. The line of weight passes in front of the knee joints even throughout normal swaying, and non-contractile structures resist further extension of the knee. Electromyographic studies confirm the lack of activity in the knee extensors and flexors during standing at ease.

Forward leaning activates the hamstrings, and backward leaning activates the quadriceps femoris to prevent flexion of the knees which would occur due to gravity.

39.   The line of weight passes behind the hip joints during standing-at-ease but the potential for extension is small. Leaning forwards activates the hamstring muscles and contraction of the abdominal muscles leads to activation of the iliopsoas muscles. During standing the hip extensors are not contracted but opinion differs with regard to the hip flexors. The close alignment of the centre of gravity of the upper body over the hip joints suggests that the hip is in equilibrium, unstable to flexion but stable to extension.

40.   The line of weight passes in front of the sacroiliac joints but forward flexion at that joint is limited by the anterior sacroiliac ligaments and the sacrospinous and sacrotuberous ligaments. Once the sacroiliac joints have been relatively immobilized by ligaments, the lower spine and pelvis move in unison. When the lower spine, pelvis and femora are stabilized the abdominal muscles act as trunk flexors and the paravertebral muscles act as trunk extensors. The hamstrings, gluteus maximus and abdominal muscles flatten the lumbar lordosis whilst the paravertebral muscles increase the lumbar lordosis.

41.   In the standing-at-ease position the line of weight passes in front of the lumbar curve and 75 per cent of subjects show activity of their erectores spinae muscles. The other 25 per cent show activity of their abdominal muscles and these electromyographic findings conform with roentgenographic and anthropometric measurements. Thus gravity tends to straighten the lumbar lordosis.

42.   The lateral muscles of the trunk laterally flex the lumbar vertebral column to the same side and rotate it contralaterally. Furthermore the psoas tends to accentuate the lumbar lordosis.

SECTION II
THE MOTION
SEGMENTS

7 Building blocks

One of the major requirements in the evolution of the spine has been flexibility without weakness. One method of imparting flexibility is by segmentation. In fish the spine is segmented thus enabling side to side movements to take place. These range from tail movements alone in some species to lateral undulations which progress along the whole animal from front to rear in others. The vertebral column of the fish can be regarded as a series of rigid units hinged to each other by surfaces that allow the body to bend only sideways. The centra of the vertebrae of most fish are concave at both ends (this arrangement also exists in less-specialized urodeles and in primitive living reptiles). In bony fish a neural arch and neural spine are associated with each vertebral centrum (Figure **7.1**). In the tail region there is also a haemal arch and haemal spine. Centra occupy the position immediately beneath the neural tube. During embryonic life the notochord occupied this position before it developed into a chain of ossified elements connected by intervening deformable discs.

The successive neural arches and associated ligaments enclose a long neural canal within which lies the spinal cord. The haemal arch encloses the caudal artery and vein. It is found not only in the tail of fish, but also in urodeles, most reptiles, some birds and many long-tailed mammals including cats.

Vertebral columns with centra concave at both ends (amphicelous centra) are extremely flexible but excessive movements must be prevented by strong ligaments. Teleosts have well-ossified amphicelous vertebrae and although the notochord persists within each centrum, it is usually very constricted. It is prominent between centra and there the notochord sheath forms strong intervertebral ligaments (Figure **7.2**).

A variety of processes protrude from the centra and arches and articulate

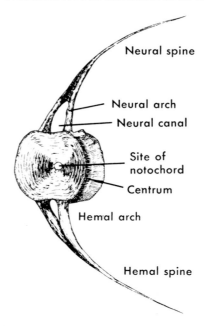

Figure 7.1   Tail vertebra of a fish (from Kent, 1973)

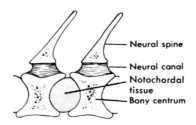

Figure 7.2   Amphicelous centra (from Kent, 1973)

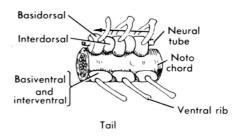

Figure 7.3   Vertebral components in adult lungfish (from Kent, 1973)

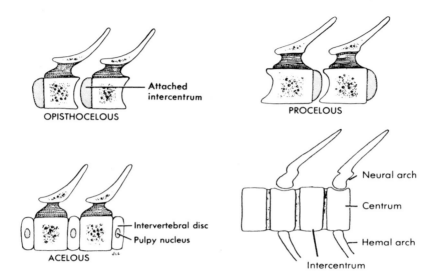

Figure 7.4 Vertebral types based on shape of articular surfaces and shown in longitudinal sections. The pulpy nucleus is a notochordal remnant (from Kent, 1973)

with similar processes on adjacent vertebrae. For the most part these processes are not comparable with those of tetrapods.

In lungfish there are no complete centra (Figure **7.3**). The notochord is unconstricted throughout its length'and cartilage provides rigidity. Lying against the notochord on each side ventrally in each segment are basiventral and interventral cartilages; perched above the notochord and forming neural arches are basidorsal and interdorsal cartilages. Kent (1973) is uncertain whether this condition is an arrested embryonic state or an extreme specialization.

Specialized urodeles have centra which are concave only on the posterior end (opisthocelous), most modern reptiles have centra which are concave only anteriorly (procelous), the centra of mammals are flat on both ends (acelous) whereas the highly flexible neck of birds has centra which are saddle-shaped at the ends (heterocelous). Many early amphibians and reptiles had an intercentrum interposed between two centra (Figure **7.4**).

None of the vertebral columns are prevented from flexing in any direction by the configuration of the centra and intervening notochordal tissues or remnants, but excessive or inappropriate movements are limited by projections from the arches and centra. These processes (or apophyses) increase the rigidity of the column and sometimes serve as the attachment for muscles. Transverse processes (diapophyses) are the most common. They are attached to the base of the neural arch or centrum and extend laterally between the dorsal and ventral muscles (Figure **7.5**).

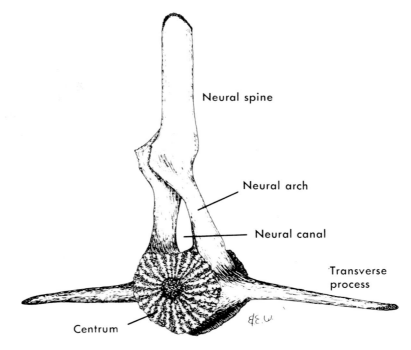

Figure 7.5   Vertebra of porpoise (from Kent, 1973)

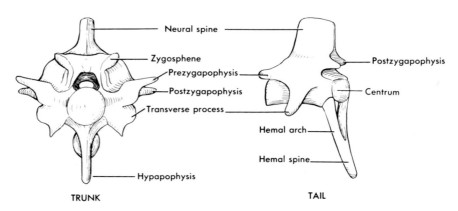

Figure 7.6   Python vertebrae; cephalic and lateral views (from Kent, 1973)

A pair of prezygapophyses frequently project cephalically from the neural arch and a pair of postzygapophyses project caudally, articulating with one another and limiting the amount of flexion/extension and torsion of the vertebral column (Figure **7.6**).

The vertebral column of the earliest tetrapods did not consist of one

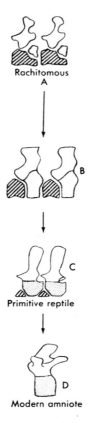

Rachitomous
A

B

Primitive reptile
C

D
Modern amniote

Figure 7.7 Modifications of tetrapod vertebrae leading to modern amniotes. The rachitomous type occurred in lobe fins and in the earliest amphibians. B is from a labyrinthodont in the reptile line (from Kent, 1973)

vertebra per body segment as it does in most tetrapods today. The 'vertebra' of the earliest amphibians consisted of a hypocentrum (intercentrum), a large anterior median wedge-shaped element that was incomplete dorsally, and two pleurocentra (smaller intersegmental posterodorsal elements). A vertebra of this kind is rachitomous. All later tetrapod vertebrae are probably modifications of the rachitomous types. Successive changes leading to modern amniotes appear to have been characterized by progressive increase in size of the pleurocentrum (Figure **7.7**).

In modern tetrapods each vertebra commences development at several loci surrounding the spinal cord and notochord. As these loci enlarge they may remain independent or unite. The typical adult vertebra is a composite structure. An adult vertebra composed of a single centrum and neural arch for each body segment is a specialized condition.

An extended series of ribs commencing immediately behind the head and

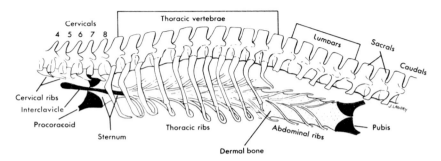

Figure 7.8   Cervical, thoracic, and vestiges of abdominal ribs (gastralia) of an alligator (from Kent, 1973)

extending into the tail facilitated locomotion via body wall muscles in fish. This was also the rib pattern in early amphibians and reptiles. As early tetrapods developed better locomotor limbs, long ribs became confined to the trunk and later to the cephalic part of the trunk. Other ribs became shortened and usually fused with the transverse processes. All the ribs in frogs are of this kind. Also in the cervical, lumbar and sacral regions of most vertebrates short vestiges of ribs are fused with transverse or other processes. Remnants of abdominal ribs have persisted in the ventral body wall of crocodilians and a few lizards (Figure **7.8**). Extra ribs in the neck or trunk occur occasionally as anomalies in many vertebrates, including man.

With the advent of terrestrial life adaptive changes occurred in the axial skeleton and the terms trunk and caudal vertebrae as applied to fish do not suffice for the tetrapod vertebral column. Tetrapod limbs push against the earth and the force is transmitted via an expanded pelvic girdle to the caudalmost trunk vertebrae. These became modified and are called sacral vertebrae. Land vertebrates also developed a flexible neck by reducing the length of the ribs of the cervical vertebrae. Amphibians were the first tetrapods to exhibit these modifications and their vertebral column consists of cervical (1), dorsal (variable number), sacral (1) and caudal (variable number) vertebrae. In crocodilians, most lizards and all birds and mammals the dorsals have become thoracic vertebrae bearing long ribs and lumbar vertebrae with ribs greatly reduced or absent.

Amphibians have a single cervical vertebra and reptiles approximately eight. The cervical region in birds is unusually flexible. This specialization is especially useful in feeding and is made possible by heterocelous vertebrae, the caudal ends of which are saddle-shaped, with a convexity in the right–left axis and a concavity in the dorsoventral axis. The cephalic end of the next centrum is shaped to accommodate this configuration. The number of cervical vertebrae varies in birds; the long neck of the swan has 25. Mammals almost always have seven cervical vertebrae. In moles several cervical vertebrae ankylose to strengthen the neck for burrowing; in marine mammals there is no external evidence of a neck region and all the cervical vertebrae are shortened and more or less fused together.

Amphibians have only one sacral vertebra and all living reptiles and most birds have only two. In birds the last thoracic, all the lumbars, the two sacrals and the first few caudal vertebrae unite to form one bone, the synsacrum. This becomes fused with the pelvic girdle. Mammals have three to five sacral vertebrae fused to form a single bony complex, the sacrum. In whales there are no hindlimbs and consequently neither pelvic girdle nor sacrum.

Primitive tetrapods had 50 or more caudal vertebrae but this number has been reduced in most mammals to approximately 20 in the horse, sheep, cat and dog, and three to five in man. Birds and mammals still have remnants of an ancestral reptilian tail and some birds retain more tail vertebrae than do some mammals.

In mammals different types of vertebrae are evident along the length of the back. The neural spines and other projections and facets gradually change in direction and in length. Young (1975) considers that the vertebral girder of the rabbit consists of two parts: lumbosacral and cervicothoracic. He believes each of these has a central main compression member (the vertebral centra) with struts on the dorsal and ventral surfaces. In the lumbosacral girder the dorsal struts are the neural spines and mamillary processes and the ventral struts are the transverse processes. In the thoracic region the dorsal struts are the neural spines and the ventral struts are the transverse processes and ribs. As the rabbit has only a small tail, the spine between its pectoral and pelvic girdles acts as a loaded beam, and its dorsal part is subject to compressive forces whilst its ventral part is subject to tensile

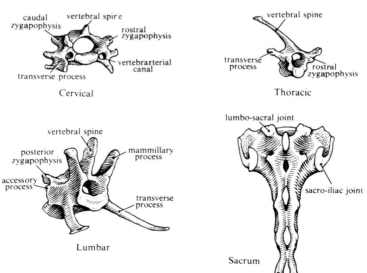

Figure 7.9 Vertebrae of a rabbit (from Young, 1975)

forces. It is worth noting that the centra, which resist the compressive forces, appear relatively dorsal in the spine on account of the large ventral transverse processes. In the dorsal region, where the spine may be said to balance like a cantilever on the forelegs, it is subject to compressive forces ventrally and to tensile forces dorsally. In this region the centra appear relatively ventral due to the very long vertebral spines (Figure **7.9**).

The maximal bending moments are in the lumbar region and here the vertebral bodies are the largest. These vertebrae allow flexion, extension and a little rotation permitting the back to arch and straighten. The more caudal of the thoracic vertebrae resemble the lumbars in some respects but whereas the lumbar transverse processes point headwards, the ribs point caudally. The neural spines also change direction just in front of this level, and the whole pattern of ties and struts alters as the system changes from the posterior loaded beam to the more anterior balanced cantilever. In the thoracic region the neural spines are extremely long and point backwards with the supraspinous ligament forming the upper tension member of the cantilever girder. In man, where the column is not constructed as a cantilever girder system, all the spines point caudally but the thoracic spines do so more sharply than the lumbar (see Figure **5.3**).

In man each typical presacral vertebra is composed of four parts:

(1) the body, which is primarily for transmission of forces
(2) the lamina and pedicles which enclose the spinal canal
(3) the spinous and transverse processes for muscle and ligament attachment
(4) the posterior facets, which guide and limit motion between vertebrae.

Kapandji (1974) has described the physiology of the joints so well that it is not possible to better his account of the structure of the typical vertebra. The vertebral body (1, Figure **7.10**) lies anteriorly and is the largest part of the

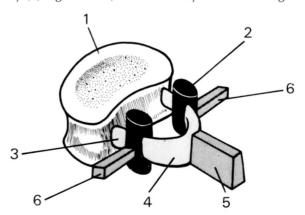

Figure 7.10   Constituents of a vertebra (see text for key) (from Kapandji, 1974)

vertebra. The vertebral arch is shaped like a horseshoe and lies behind the vertebral body. It bears on each side an articular process (2), which divides the arch into an anterior pedicle (3) and a posterior lamina (4). The spinous process (5) is attached to the midline posteriorly. The vertebral arch therefore is attached to the vertebral body by the pedicles. Transverse processes (6) are attached to the arch near the articular processes.

In the vertical plane these various constituents lie in anatomical correspondence making three pillars: an anterior, major pillar comprising the stacked vertebral bodies, and two posterior, minor pillars made up of the articular processes (Figure **7.11**).

The vertebral body has a dense bony cortex surrounding a spongy medulla. The cortex of the superior and inferior aspects is called the vertebral plateau. The periphery is thickened to form a distinct rim which is derived from the epiphyseal plate and becomes fused to the body at 14–15 years of age (Figure **7.12**). A section of the vertebra taken in the verticofrontal plane shows the thick cortex on either side, the cartilage-lined vertebral plateau superiorly and inferiorly, and the spongy centre of the

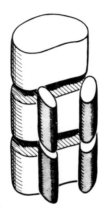

Figure 7.11   The three anatomical pillars (from Kapandji, 1974)

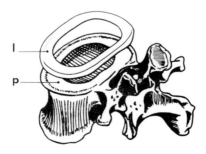

Figure 7.12   Vertebral plateau (p) and rim (l) (from Kapandji, 1974)

vertebral body with bony trabeculae disposed along the lines of force (Figure **7.13**). These lines are vertical linking the superior and inferior surfaces, horizontal linking the lateral surfaces, and oblique linking the inferior and lateral surfaces. The sagittal section shows in addition two fan-like sheaves of oblique fibres. The first, arising from the superior surface,

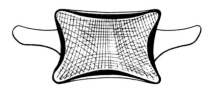

Figure 7.13   Section of vertebra in verticofrontal plane (from Kapandji, 1974)

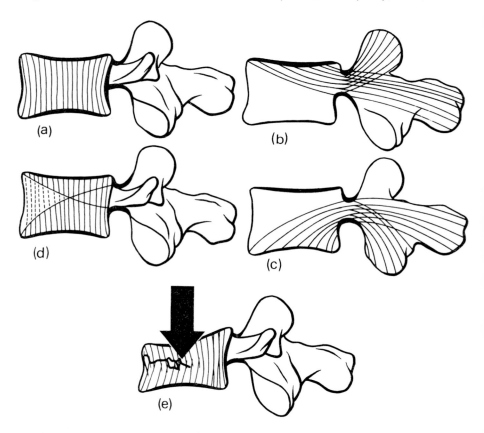

Figure 7.14   Lines of force of vertebra showing triangle in (d) of minimum resistance which leads to wedge-shaped compression fracture shown in (e) (from Kapandji, 1974)

fans out at the level of the two pedicles to reach the corresponding superior articular processes and spinous process. The second, arising from the inferior surface, fans out at the level of the two pedicles to reach the corresponding inferior articular processes and spinous process. The criss-crossing of these three trabecular systems constitutes zones of maximum resistance as well as a triangular area of minimum resistance. This triangle is made up only of vertical trabeculae and explains the wedge-shaped compression fractures that occur (Figure **7.14**).

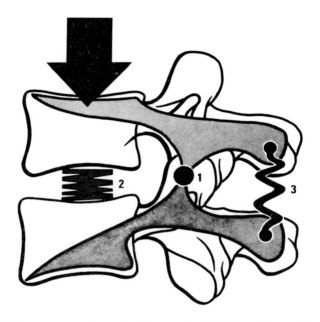

Figure 7.15 Lever system of vertebra (see text for key) (from Kapandji, 1974)

Each vertebra can be compared to a lever system where the articular processes (1, Figure **7.15**) constitute the fulcrum. This lever system allows the absorption of axial compression forces applied to the vertebral bodies (2), and indirect absorption in the posterior ligaments and muscles (3).

The superior articular process (1, Figure **7.16**) of a lumbar vertebra lies in a plane such that its cartilage-lined articular surface faces posteriorly and medially. The inferior articular process (2) has an articular surface which faces laterally and anteriorly. This configuration allows a certain degree of anteroposterior and lateral flexion between adjacent lumbar vertebrae, but rotation about a perpendicular through the centres of the vertebral plateaux is prevented (Figure **7.17**).

The profiles of the lumbar superior articular processes correspond to a

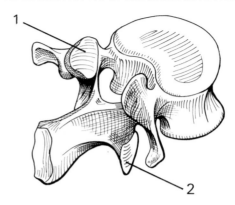

Figure 7.16 Superior articular process (1) and inferior articular process (2) of vertebra (from Kapandji, 1974)

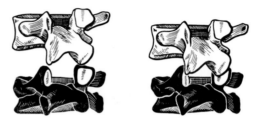

Figure 7.17 Prevention of rotation by articular processes (from Kapandji, 1974)

cylinder with centre O located posteriorly near the base of the spinous process (Figure **7.18**). In the lower lumbar vertebrae the diameter of this cylinder is comparatively greater. The centre of this cylinder does not coincide with the centre of the vertebral plateaux so when the upper vertebra rotates on the lower one the upper vertebra's body must slide over that of the lower vertebra. The shearing forces that ensue limit the rotation so that it is minimal both segmentally and over the whole lumbar spine.

The typical thoracic vertebra is made up of the same parts as a lumbar vertebra but there are structural and functional differences. The vertebral body is proportionately taller than that of lumbar vertebrae and its anterior and lateral surfaces are quite hollow. The oval facet of the superior articular process faces posteriorly, slightly superiorly and slightly laterally. The oval facet of the inferior articular process faces anteriorly, slightly inferiorly and medially (Figure **7.19**).

Although the superior articular processes of the twelfth thoracic vertebra resemble those of the other thoracic vertebrae, the inferior articular processes must correspond to those of L_1 so they face laterally and anteriorly. The thoracic vertebrae allow a certain amount of forward flexion,

UPPER LUMBAR   LOWER LUMBAR

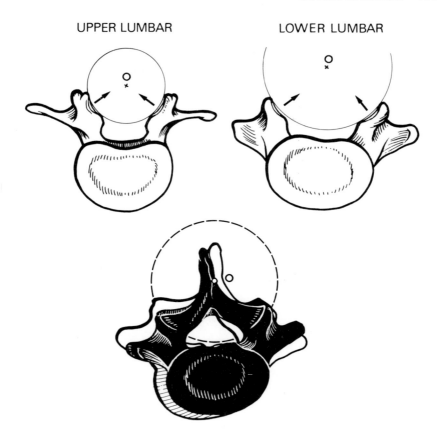

Figure 7.18 Centres of rotation of cylinders passing through articular processes of lumbar vertebrae showing generation of shearing forces during rotation. (from Kapandji, 1974)

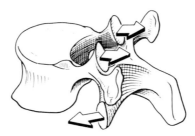

Figure 7.19 Planes of articular processes of thoracic vertebrae are consistent with *rotation* between vertebrae (from Kapandji, 1974)

extension and lateral flexion to take place at each intervertebral level but the thoracic column is connected to the thoracic cage by multiple joints, and all components of the cage play a role in orientating and limiting the basic movement of the column. The mechanism of axial rotation at thoracic level differs from that seen at the lumbar level. The profile of the facet joints also corresponds to the surface of a cylinder but the centre of this cylinder lies nearer the centre of each vertebral body. Davies (1959) has studied the medial inclination of the thoracic intervertebral articular facets and concluded that simple rotation can occur in the midthoracic region, but elsewhere in the thoracic spine rotation must be accompanied by a lateral shearing of the bodies because the centre of the cylinder lies in front of the vertebral bodies. When one vertebra rotates on another, the articular facets slide relative to each other but the rotation is limited by the attachment of the thoracic column with the remainder of the bony thorax. When the thorax is still flexible, as in the young, the movements of the thoracic column have a considerable range but with age the costal cartilages ossify and movement is reduced.

IN SUMMARY

43. Segmentation allowed the spine to remain flexible in spite of becoming bony. The notochord developed into a chain of ossified elements connected by intervening deformable discs.

44. The ossified elements or vertebral centra are flat at both ends in mammals though concave on at least one end in other vertebrates.

45. In fish it is possible to distinguish only trunk and caudal vertebrae. In quadrupeds the caudalmost trunk vertebrae became modified to withstand the force generated through the hindlimbs – sacral vertebrae. Land vertebrates also developed a flexible neck by reducing the length of the ribs of the cervical vertebrae.

46. The remaining trunk vertebrae are either thoracic or lumbar. In mammals only the thoracic vertebrae articulate with ribs. Mammals almost always have seven cervical vertebrae, nine to 25 thoracic vertebrae, five to eight lumbar vertebrae, three to five sacral vertebrae, and three to 50 caudal vertebrae.

47. Projections from the neural arches and centra increase the rigidity of the column. These processes limit the amount of movement between vertebrae and serve as the attachment for muscles. The shape and size of the processes differ in various regions along the length of the back.

48. The centra and articular processes of the human spine constitute three vertical pillars. The centra contain bony trabeculae along the lines of force. In addition two fan-like sheaves pass from the vertebral plateaux to the articular processes.

49.   The system allows absorption of axial compression forces directly in the vertebral bodies and indirectly in the posterior ligaments and muscles.
50.   The articular surfaces of the lumbar apophyseal joints allow anterior flexion, extension and lateral flexion but not rotation about a line through the centra. The corresponding joints of the thoracic vertebrae allow flexion, extension, lateral flexion and rotation. The anatomical pattern suggests that rotation is possible maximally in the mid-thoracic region.

8 Spinal mobility

The structure of the vertebrae determines to a large extent the mechanics of the spinal column. We have seen that a particularly important anatomical variation which modifies the spinal movement at any one level is the structure of adjacent articular processes of apophyseal joints. The contact established between the superior articular processes of one vertebra and the inferior articular processes of the next stabilizes vertebral movement and in particular prevents forward displacement of one vertebra on another. The angle of the articular surfaces of the apophyseal joints in relation to the horizontal plane of the vertebral bodies varies at different levels, and largely determines the type as well as the amount of movement occurring at various levels of the spine. Moll and Wright (1971) remind us that movement between adjacent vertebrae is maximal at spinal levels where the disc is thickest, as in the cervical and lumbar regions, and least where the disc is thinnest, as in the thoracic region. The dense anterior longitudinal ligament is stronger than the posterior ligament and limits extension of the vertebral column. The ligamenta flava help to restore the vertebral column to its original position after bending movements, and White and Hirsch (1971) emphasize their importance in resisting rotation. The spinous processes are connected by the supraspinous and interspinous ligaments which particularly limit flexion.

The spinal column has three degrees of freedom; it is allowed flexion and extension, lateral flexion and rotation. The range of these elementary movements at each individual joint is very small, but the movements are cumulative over the whole column. Moll and Wright found an initial increase in mean spinal mobility from the 15–24 decade to the 25–34 decade followed by a progressive decrease with advancing age of as much as 50 per cent of mobility. The scatter of spinal mobility varied between decades, but

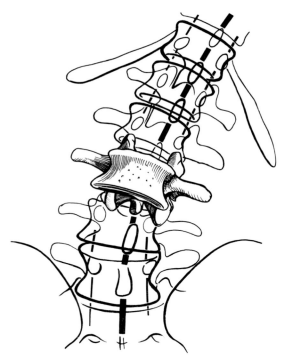

Figure 8.1   Rotation which occurs during lateral flexion (from Kapandji, 1974)

in each age group it was considerable. The wide range of normal mobility was seen in flexion, extension and lateral flexion. A sex difference was observed at each decade in all three planes of movement. In anterior flexion and extension, male mobility exceeded female mobility, whereas in lateral flexion the converse was observed. Other workers have found different patterns of spinal mobility between the sexes. Isdale (1976) has found all spinal movements to be greater in the female. Sturrock, Wojtulewski, and Hart (1973) found female anterior flexion to exceed that in males although the male extension was greater than female extension.

Kapandji (1974) quotes segmental contributions to flexion and extension measured from radiographs as 60° flexion and 35° extension at the lumbar level. For the thoracolumbar region taken as a whole, flexion is maximally 105° and extension 60°.

Of the 90° or so of combined lumbar flexion and extension, 22 per cent takes place between L_5 and S_1, 29 per cent between L_4 and L_5, 22 per cent between L_3 and L_4, 14 per cent between L_2 and L_3, and 13 per cent takes place between L_1 and L_2. According to Tanz (1950 and 1953) the range of flexion decreases with age being maximal between 2 and 13 years of age.

Again using radiographs Kapandji gives the ranges of lateral flexion to each side as 20° in the lumbar column and 20° in the thoracic column.

Of the 20° of lumbar lateral flexion 6 per cent takes place between L_5 and S_1, 26 per cent between L_4 and L_5, 26 per cent between L_3 and L_4, 26 per cent between L_2 and L_3, and 16 per cent takes place between L_1 and L_2. Lateral flexion between L_5 and S_1 is limited by the strong inferior iliolumbar ligaments.

During lateral flexion the vertebral bodies rotate contralaterally. This rotation can be seen on anteroposterior radiographs: the bodies lose their symmetry and the interspinous line moves towards the side of movement (Figure **8.1**).

Loebl (1973) has reported normal values for thoracolumbar rotation of 67° in the thoracic spine and 25° in the lumbar spine. These correlate well with Beetham *et al.* (1966) who quote figures of 90° of rotation to either side for the 'trunk' and 30° to either side for the 'lower thoracic and lumbar

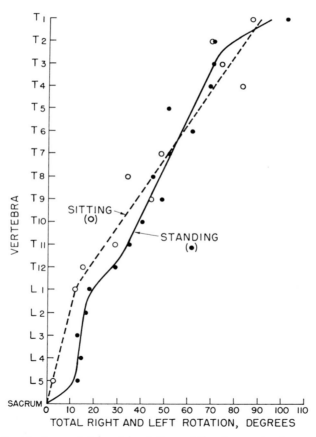

Figure 8.2 Maximum total axial rotation of the thoracolumbar spine in the standing and sitting positions (pelvis immobilized) (from Gregersen and Lucas, 1967)

segments'. The work of Gregersen and Lucas (1967) has provided accurate measurements. Under general anaesthesia they implanted metal pins into the spinous processes of the thoracic and lumbar vertebrae and measured their displacements telemetrically. They were thus able to measure rotation of the thoracolumbar column during walking, standing and sitting (Figure **8.2**).

The subjects (standing erect, then sitting, with axial rotation measured relative to the fixed pelvis) turned from side to side as far as possible. In one subject, 9° of rotation occurred between the first and the fifth lumbar vertebrae during standing and 8° during sitting; additional rotation of approximately 10° was observed at the thoracolumbar joint. An average of approximately 6° was measured at each of the remaining thoracic levels.

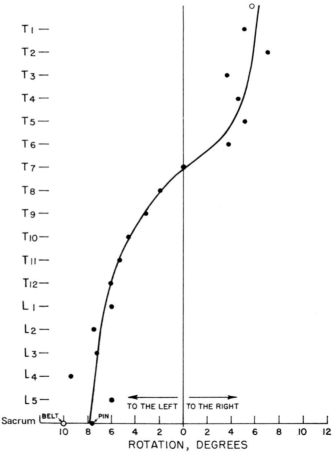

Figure 8.3 Axial rotation of the thoracolumbar spine during locomotion (left heel strike to right heel strike, 4.38 km/h) (from Gregersen and Lucas, 1967)

Some individual variation in the amount of axial rotation was observed in the subjects tested. In one half of a walking cycle during normal level walking on a treadmill, 5° of rotation occurred at the first thoracic vertebra and, in the opposite direction 6° at the fifth lumbar vertebra. There appeared to be a transition point (displacement node) in the sixth to eighth thoracic vertebral region above which rotation was in the direction opposite to that below (Figure **8.3**). Next to this pivotal interspace relative rotation is greatest but it progressively decreases upwards and downwards to become minimal in the lumbar and upper thoracic regions (Figure **8.4**).

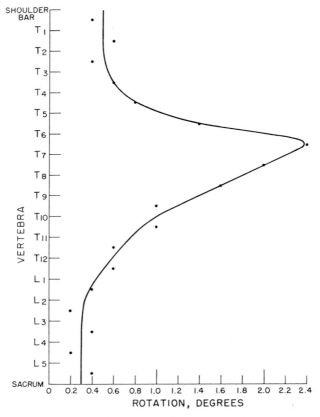

Figure 8.4 Axial rotation between adjacent vertebrae during locomotion (4.38 km/h) (derived from curve of Figure 8.3) (from Gregersen and Lucas, 1967)

Gregersen and Lucas investigated the effect on their subjects of carrying a 4.5 kg (10 lb) weight in each hand during walking. It appeared that the normal pattern of rotation, with change in direction at a nodal point in the middle of the thoracic spine, was altered by the damping effect of the addition of weights on arm swing and the node shifted upward to a higher

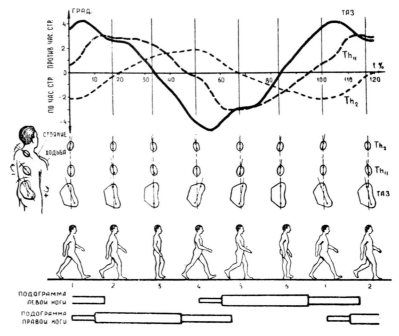

Figure 8.5   Axial rotation of shoulder girdle and pelvis during walking (from Belenky, 1971)

point in the thoracic spine. In an additional study, axial rotation was found to occur with motion of the spine in the coronal plane, an observation that supports the concept that axial rotation is an integral motion of the thoracolumbar spine during lateral bending.

Although for the sitting and standing positions the degree of rotation observed by Gregersen and Lucas was less than that observed by other workers, axial rotation of the thoracolumbar column was consistently greatest in the mid-thoracic region. This finding is in harmony with the planes of the articular surfaces of the apophyseal joints. Belenky (1971) writes that axial rotation of the vertebrae is not only determined by the inter-position of the pelvis and shoulder girdle, but also appears to depend on the changing rigidity of the muscle sheath surrounding the spine. This observation resulted from a study of movements of the pelvis and spine during walking in 16 normal subjects. Rotation of the pelvis and vertebrae was measured with the aid of a free gyroscope, and a record of displace-ments of the vertebrae in relation to the pelvis was obtained by a special device equipped with tensometric pick-ups (Figure **8.5**).

We have, therefore, seen locomotion generated by a side to side movement of the spine in fish and swimming amphibians. When animals became wholly terrestrial the lateral undulations of the spine were replaced

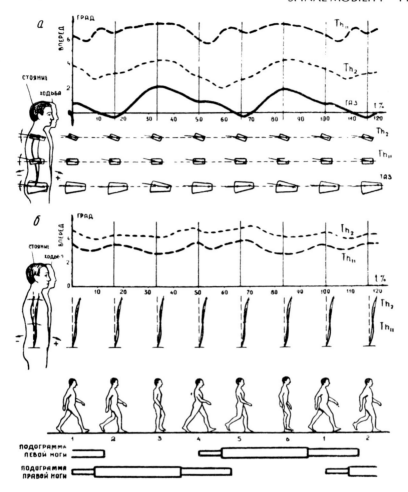

Figure 8.6 Flattening of natural curves of spine during walking (from Belenky, 1971)

largely by movement powered by the limbs. In some quadrupeds limb locomotion is aided by anterior flexion/extension of the spine which increases the span between footfalls. Even in man anterior flexion/extension of the thoracolumbar spine occurs during walking and this takes place primarily in the lumbar region. Belenky showed that the spine in the sagittal plane during walking is thrust forward slightly with flattening of its natural curves. Together with the pelvis, it effectuates mild swing motions (Figure **8.6**).

Belenky also measured the side to side movements of the spine during walking. He found the rotary motions in the frontal plane of the spine to be of the same order of magnitude as those of the pelvis, but opposite in direction. This helps to maintain the body in a vertical position during the process of propulsion. Nevertheless displacement of the thoracic and lumbar segments at various phases in the walking cycle are not identical and the entire spine assumes either an S-curve or a C-curve. He simplifies this

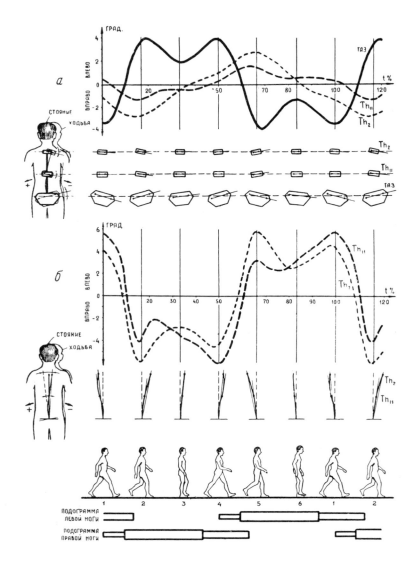

Figure 8.7   Side-to-side movements of the spine during walking (from Belenky, 1971)

picture by saying that movements of the lumbar spine neutralize the tilts of the pelvis, while displacements of the thoracic spine favour deviation of the centre of gravity to the side of the weight-bearing leg (Figure **8.7**)

Napier (1967) reminds us that the human stride demands both an up-and-down and a side to side displacement of the body. When two people walk side by side but out of step, the alternate bobbing of their heads makes it evident that the bodies undergo a vertical displacement with each stride. When two people walk in step but with opposite feet leading, they will sway first toward each other and then away in an equally graphic demonstration of the lateral displacement at each stride. When both displacements are plotted sequentially, a pair of low-amplitude sinusoidal curves appear, one in the vertical plane and the other in the horizontal.

The pelvis plays an important role in walking; its degree of rotation in the horizontal plane determines the distance the swinging leg can move forward. The difference in the proportions of the male and the female pelvis has the effect of slightly diminishing the range through which the female hip can move forward and back, and we have noted already that women are obliged to rotate the pelvis through a greater angle than do men. This secondary sexual characteristic has not lacked exploitation.

Pelvic rotation during walking without an equal and opposite rotation higher in the spine would lead to rotation of the head and shoulders from one side to the other with each step. All hunting animals have mechanisms for stabilizing the plane of their eyes whilst stalking, and perhaps man maintains his head directed to the front for the same reason. Alternatively the damping of the pelvic rotation might be an energy-saving mechanism which developed at the same time as man's striding gait and allowed him to cover large distances on foot. Whatever the reason the result of head (and shoulder) stability is achieved by swinging the arms during walking to rotate the shoulder girdle in the opposite direction to the rotation of the pelvis. During normal walking Ballesteros (1965) has estimated the forward swing of the arms to be 20° and the backward swing about 9°. The former is brought about by some of the inward rotators rather than by the flexors; the latter by some of the extensors and outward rotators. The arm swing tends to be slightly across the body. This is exaggerated if the individual is short and broad-shouldered. The sideways movement of the arms helps to compensate for the sideways movement of the body.

Axial rotation in the spine was possible only after the change to a bipedal gait enabled the shoulder girdle to rotate independently of the pelvis. This rotation takes place maximally in the mid-thoracic region where the inclinations of the intervertebral articular facets permit rotation without shearing of the vertebral bodies. Telemetric studies confirm that rotation is greatest at the T_7–T_8 level during walking. Thus as well as side to side movements of the spine and flexion/extension, man has added movement in the third dimension to assist with his locomotion—axial rotation.

IN SUMMARY

51. The lumbar spine contributes 60° of forward flexion and 35° of extension to spinal mobility. For the thoracolumbar region taken as a whole, flexion is maximally 105° and extension 60°. Of the 90° or so of combined lumbar flexion and extension, the ratio that takes place between L_5 and S_1, L_4 and L_5, L_3 and L_4, L_2 and L_3, L_1 and L_2 is 3:4:3:2:2.

52. The range of lateral flexion to each side is 20° in the lumbar column and a further 20° in the thoracic column. Of the 20° of lumbar flexion the ratio that takes place between L_1 and S_1, L_4 and L_5, L_3 and L_4, L_2 and L_3, L_1 and L_2 is 1:4:4:4:3. During lateral flexion the vertebral bodies rotate contralaterally and the interspinous line moves towards the side of movement.

53. The range of axial rotation from side to side during standing is 20° in the lumbar column and 90° for the thoracolumbar region taken as a whole; 10° takes place at the thoracolumbar joint.

54. During normal walking 5° of axial rotation takes place at the first thoracic vertebra and, in the opposite direction, 6° at the fifth lumbar vertebra. The node of transition lies in the sixth to eighth thoracic vertebral region. Adjacent to this pivotal interspace relative rotation is greatest and it progressively decreases upwards and downwards. Carrying a 4.5 kg (10 lb) weight in each hand during walking moves the node to a higher point in the thoracic spine.

55. During walking the spine is thrust forward in the sagittal plane with flattening of its natural curves. These movements damp the up-and-down displacement of the body but the head still follows a residual, low-amplitude sinusoidal path. There is a similar side to side displacement of the trunk during walking which favours deviation of the centre of gravity to the weight-bearing leg. This is produced by displacements of the thoracic spine while the lumbar spine tends to neutralize the tilts of the pelvis.

56. The pelvic axial rotation during walking is damped by arm-swinging which rotates the shoulder girdle in an opposite direction to that of the pelvis. This rotation takes place maximally in the mid-thoracic region.

9

The role of the discs

The extensive degree of mobility of the thoracolumbar spine described in the last chapter is possible only because the spine in this region is segmented into 17 separate vertebrae. This mobility, and the need for simultaneous load-bearing, necessitates some form of hydrostatic structure to convert unidirectional forces into stresses acting in all directions. Several authors, including Schmorl (1926), Beadle (1931), and Shah (1976) have considered the nucleus pulposus of the intervertebral disc to be a perfect hydrostatic medium. It distributes the axial load radially to be absorbed by the fibres of the surrounding annulus fibrosus. Macnab (1977) has compared this function of the annulus to the hoops around a barrel.

The hydrostatic action of the nucleus was predicted because of its high water content, but was not proven experimentally until Nachemson punctured the nucleus pulposus in 1960 with a specially constructed hollow needle connected to an electromanometer. He related the forces acting in the nucleus to the forces acting in the annulus. When a vertebral plateau presses on the intervertebral disc the nucleus bears 75 per cent of the force and the annulus 25 per cent. The nucleus transmits some of the force to the annulus in the horizontal plane and the tangential tensile strain is four to five times the applied external load.

Incarcerated under pressure within its casing between two vertebral plateaux, the nucleus pulposus is roughly spherical; Kapandji (1974) likens it to a ball between two parallel planes. The pressure in the centre of the ball is never zero, even when the disc is unloaded. This preloaded state provides greater resistance to the forces of compression and to lateral flexion. Virgin (1951) noted the intrinsic pressure in the discs of cadaver spines and Nachemson and Evans (1968) later demonstrated that the ligamentum flavum, situated between the posterior arches and facets, prestresses the disc and provides some intrinsic stability to the spine. The intrinsic pressure is due to the water-absorbing capacity of the disc. With age the nucleus loses its water-absorbing capacity and the preloaded state tends to be lost; hence the lack of flexibility of the vertebral column in the aged. During standing the water in the gelatinous matrix of the nucleus escapes into the vertebral body through microscopic pores and during the course of the day the disc becomes thinner. At night the water-absorbing capacity of the nucleus draws water back into the nucleus from the vertebral bodies and the disc regains its original thickness. Therefore flexibility of the vertebral column is greatest in the morning and at this time the spine is longer than in the evening.

The notochord constitutes the earliest structure to stiffen the embryo, appearing in animals before the true vertebral column develops. In lungfish the notochord remains unconstricted throughout its length and cartilage imparts rigidity to it. In Agnatha the notochord and its sheath persist throughout life although rudimentary neural arches are found in the adult lamprey. Modern sharks possess a vertebral column composed of cartilaginous centra that have their origin within the sheath of the notochord, thus causing its partial absorption. Among the bony fish the sturgeon has a persistent notochord with a fibrous sheath on which paired cartilaginous arches appear. The vertebrae of the more advanced bony fish are completely ossified. In reptiles fibrocartilaginous intervertebral discs, or intercentra, unite the centra whereas in mammals the vertebral centra articulate by means of intervertebral discs of fibrocartilage. The pulpy nucleus of the disc is a notochordal remnant and the vertebral column is formed around the notochordal framework. The notochord can still be identified for some time traversing the cartilaginous centra but these parts ultimately atrophy and vanish. Between the vertebrae, the nucleus pulposus of the intervertebral disc is surrounded by the annulus fibrosus which differentiates into an external laminated fibrous zone and an internal cuff around the nucleus. After the sixth month of human fetal life the notochordal cells in the nucleus pulposus commence to degenerate, being replaced by cells from the internal zone of the annulus fibrosus. This degeneration continues until the second decade of life by which time all the notochordal cells have disappeared. *Gray's Anatomy* (1973) tells us that in the adult, notochordal vestiges are limited, at the most, to non-cellular matrix.

As the mucoid material of the nucleus pulposus is gradually replaced by fibrocartilage in the second decade, the nucleus becomes more and more difficult to differentiate from the remainder of the disc. At birth, the water content of the annulus fibrosus is about 80 per cent and of the nucleus pulposus about 90 per cent. Vernon-Roberts (1976) states that by the third decade, the annulus contains about 70 per cent water and the nucleus about 75 per cent. Thereafter, the annulus retains a relatively constant water content of about 70 per cent, whereas the water content of the nucleus diminishes progressively to approach that of the annulus.

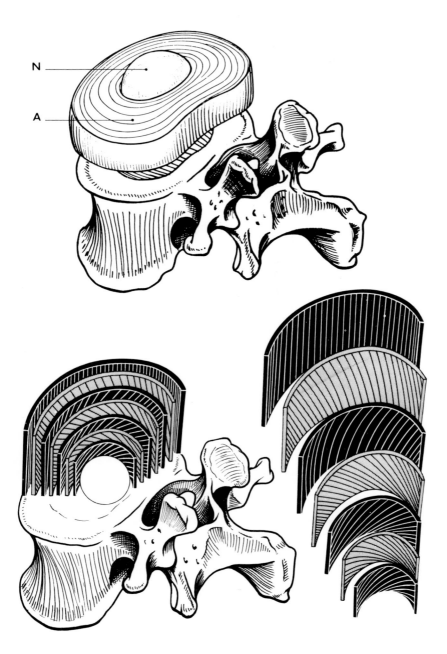

Figure 9.1   Fibres of the annulus fibrosus (A) enclosing the nucleus pulposus (N) (from Kapandji, 1974)

Kapandji (1974) describes the annulus fibrosus as made up of concentric fibres which appear to cross one another obliquely, but the fibres are vertical peripherally and become more oblique towards the centre. The central fibres in contact with the nucleus are nearly horizontal running between the vertebral plateaux in ellipsoidal fashion (Figure **9.1**). Thus the nucleus is enclosed within an inextensible casing formed by the vertebral plateaux and the annulus, whose woven fibres in the young prevent any prolapse of the nucleus.

Macnab (1977) has likened the annulus to a coiled spring, pulling the vertebral bodies together against the elastic resistance of the nucleus pulposus (Figure **9.2**).

The ensuing mobile joint allows not only flexion, extension, lateral flexion and rotation but also gliding in the horizontal plane forwards, backwards and to both sides. Macnab regards the nucleus pulposus as a ball-bearing with the vertebral bodies rolling over the incompressible gel in flexion and extension while the posterior joints guide and steady the movement. During extension the upper vertebra moves posteriorly reducing the interspace posteriorly and driving the nucleus anteriorly. The nucleus presses on the anterior fibres of the annulus increasing their tension and this tends to restore the upper vertebra to its normal position. During flexion the upper vertebra moves anteriorly reducing the interspace anteriorly and driving the nucleus posteriorly. The nucleus now presses on the posterior fibres of the annulus increasing their tension. Once more there is a self-stabilization. During axial rotation the central fibres of the annulus

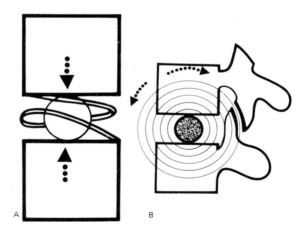

Figure 9.2 A, The annulus acts like a coiled spring, pulling the vertebral bodies together against the elastic resistance of the nucleus pulposus. B, the nucleus pulposus acts as a ball bearing with the vertebral bodies rolling over this incompressible gel in flexion and extension while the posterior joints guide and steady the movement (from Macnab, 1977)

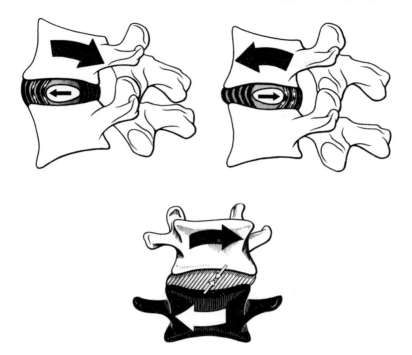

Figure 9.3 Extension, flexion and axial rotation increasing the internal disc pressure and stretching the annulus (from Kapandji, 1974)

(which are the most oblique) are stretched, compressing the nucleus and causing the internal pressure to rise. Flexion and axial rotation tend to tear the annulus and drive the nucleus posteriorly through tears in the annulus. Whatever force is applied to the disc, the internal pressure is increased and the fibres of the annulus are stretched. Owing to the relative movement of the nucleus, the stretching of the annulus tends to oppose this movement (Figure **9.3**).

The hydrostatic properties of the nucleus and the relatively high pressure that it exhibits relieves the annulus fibrosus from vertical stress, thus making tilting movements of the loaded lumbar spine easier. Nachemson (1976) showed that moderate degenerative changes in the disc, irrespective of age, do not seem to alter this mechanism. Severe degeneration is associated with a loss of the hydrostatic behaviour and a decrease of the stresses noted in the nucleus pulposus. In this case the mechanism of the disc is entirely altered.

Other tissues besides the discs are affected by these movements. During extension the upper vertebra tilts and moves backwards in the direction of the arrow E (Figure **9.4**). The anterior longitudinal ligament (5) is stretched and the posterior longitudinal ligament is relaxed. The articular processes of

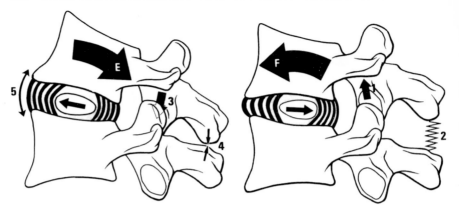

Figure 9.4   Extension (E) and flexion (F) affecting other aspects of the intervertebral joint (see text for key) (from Kapandji, 1974)

the lower and upper vertebrae become tightly interlocked (3), and the spinous processes touch one another (4). Hence to help the disc limit extension the bony structures of the vertebral arch impact and the anterior longitudinal ligament develops tension. During flexion the upper vertebra moves anteriorly in the direction of the arrow F. The inferior articular processes of the upper vertebra slide superiorly and tend to move away from the superior articular processes of the lower vertebra. As a result the ligaments of the joints between these articular processes are maximally stretched as well as all the ligaments of the vertebral arch – the ligamentum flavum, the interspinous ligament (2), the supraspinous ligament and the posterior longitudinal ligament. These stretched ligaments finally limit flexion.

During lateral flexion the intertransverse ligament on the flexed side relaxes and the opposite ligament is stretched. The articular processes slide relative to each other with stretching of the ligamenta flava and the capsular ligaments. Lateral flexion is limited by the impact of the articular processes on the side of movement and also by the stretched contralateral ligamenta flava and intertransverse ligaments.

Nachemson used his *in vitro* experiments as a basis for *in vivo* ones to study the effect of different static positions of the body on the disc pressure. Changes were observed in the third lumbar disc of a 70 kg (154 lb) subject and expressed as percentages of the pressure in the upright standing position (Figure **9.5**).

He also studied relative change in pressure in the same lumbar disc with various movements and exercises. Although standing increases the load on the disc fourfold compared to the supine position, relatively common movements like the traditional 'back-strengthening exercises' almost double the load in the disc over the standing position. Thus the gravitational effect on

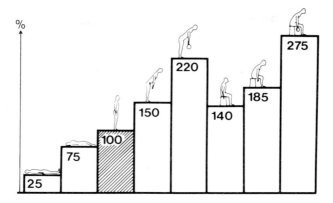

Figure 9.5   Relative change in pressure (or load) in the third lumbar disc in various positions in living subjects. This graphic evaluation clarifies the importance of both correct posture and intermittent rest (from Nachemson, 1976)

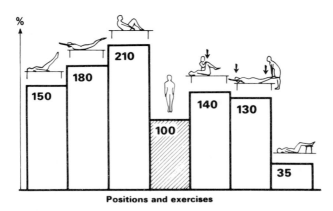

Figure 9.6   Relative change in pressure (or load) in the third lumbar disc with various muscle-strengthening exercises in living subjects. Traditional exercises and their effect on discal pressure are analysed in this table. The dangers of isotonic (so-called Williams) flexion and extension exercises are clearly demonstrated while isometric or resisted exercises give less strain to the spine (from Nachemson, 1976)

the spinal tissues of standing is overshadowed by the effect of muscular activity (Figure **9.6**).

Table 9.1 shows intradiscal pressure resulting from different activities. Beadle (1931), reporting on the original studies of Schmorl (1926), first proposed that a compressive load acting on the nucleus pulposus was the mechanical basis of disc degeneration. Other investigators devised mechanical experiments to support this hypothesis but were not able to prove that mechanical compression played a significant role in the aetiology of disc degeneration. Although they were able to show that on pure

Table 9.1   Approximate load on L_3 disc in 70 kg (154 lb) individual in different postures, movements and manoeuvres (from Nachemson (1976)

Activity	Load (kg)
Supine in traction (30 kg)	10
Supine	30
Standing	70
Walking	85
Twisting	90
Bending sideways	95
Upright sitting, no support	100
Coughing	110
Jumping	110
Isometric abdominal muscle exercise	110
Straining	120
Laughing	120
Bilateral straight leg raising, supine	120
Bending forward 20°	120
Active back hyperextension, prone	150
Sit-up exercise with knees extended	175
Sit-up exercise with knees bent	180
Bending forward 20° with 10 kg (22 lb) in each hand	185
Lifting of 20 kg (44 lb), back straight, knees bent	210
Lifting of 20 kg (44 lb), back bent, knees straight	340

vertical compression the vertebral end-plates will be the first structures to fracture, with a resulting herniation of the nucleus pulposus into the vertebral body, they were unable to produce the sort of disc hernias seen in patients. Realizing that the disc was able to support large compressive loads, it was suggested that the disc may be sensitive to torsion or bending. Farfan and Sullivan (1967) suggested that one of the functions of the joints between the articular processes was to protect the disc from excessive torsion. In a subsequent communication, Farfan (1969) showed that a twisting force was capable of producing damage to the intervertebral joint and that the joints between the articular processes did act as a protective mechanism. Furthermore, it was shown that the compressive load of body weight augmented this protective function of the articular processes rendering the whole intervertebral joint more resistant to torsion. Farfan et al. (1970) then showed that the disc of an intact lumbar intervertebral joint supplied 35 per cent of the resistance to experimentally applied torque, while the remaining 65 per cent of the resistance could be attributed to the posterior assembly comprising the articular processes, their capsules, and the interspinous ligaments. The contribution of the disc must depend on the annulus since the nucleus, being a gel, can provide little or no resistance to torsion. The condition of the annulus is therefore important and damage to it must have serious consequences on the whole joint. It is not surprising that the first signs of disc degeneration, which are often overlooked, are in the annulus. Disc rupture, induced experimentally by torsion, produced changes similar to those seen in naturally occurring disc degeneration suggesting that both changes were the result of the same causative mechanism. Farfan postulated that *in vivo* disc degeneration is due to imposed torsional strains rather than to compressive loads. Since the joints between the articular processes stabilize the intervertebral joint against torsion, he suggested that any impairment of the function of the joints between the articular processes might result in a higher risk of disc degeneration.

IN SUMMARY

57. Because of the need for both mobility and load-bearing by the thoracolumbar spine, sometimes simultaneously, some form of hydrostatic structure is needed to convert unidirectional forces into stresses acting in all directions.

58. The nucleus pulposus of the intervertebral disc fulfils this role, distributing the axial load to the fibres of the annulus fibrosus. This action is made possible by the high water content of the nucleus which helps to impart an intrinsic pressure to the disc.

59. By the second decade all the notochordal cells have disappeared from the nucleus pulposus, the mucoid material is being replaced by fibrocartilage and the water content has been reduced from 90 per cent to 75 per cent. The preloaded state becomes lost and the vertebral column becomes less flexible.

60. The nucleus pulposus can be regarded as a ball-bearing with the vertebral bodies rolling over the incompressible gel while the posterior joints guide and steady the movement. Moderate degenerative changes in the disc do not seem to alter this mechanism. Severe degeneration is associated with a loss of the hydrostatic behaviour and the mechanism of the disc is entirely altered.

61. Although standing increases the load on the disc fourfold compared to the supine position, 20° forward leaning increases the load on the disc by 50 per cent over the standing position, and 20° forward leaning with a 20 kg (44 lb) load in the hands more than doubles the load over the standing position.

62. Walking, twisting, and sideways bending are less pressure-inducing than coughing, straining and jumping. Relatively common movements like the traditional 'back-strengthening exercises' almost double the load on the disc over the standing position. It is immediately apparent that muscular activity imparts to the disc far greater loads than that presented by the effect of gravity in the standing position.

63.   Various workers have shown that on vertical compression the vertebral end-plates are the first structures to fracture and they have been unable to produce the sort of disc hernias seen in patients. Disc rupture induced experimentally by torsion produced changes similar to those seen in naturally occurring disc degeneration, suggesting that both changes were the result of the same causative mechanism.

64.   Farfan postulates that since the joints between the articular processes stabilize the intervertebral joint against torsion, any impairment of the function of the joints between the articular processes might result in a higher risk of disc degeneration.

10 Stability and strength

In Section I the human spine was treated as if it were a relatively immobile structure like a rigid rod. Early in Section II the concept of movement was introduced and the relationships of various parts of the moving spine to each other were described. This mobility was achieved by segmentation, which brought with it the need for stability. Morris (1973) writes of the intrinsic spinal stability as provided by the intervertebral discs and ligaments, and extrinsic stability imparted to the vertebral column by the action of muscles. The intrinsic stability is the result of pressure within the discs which tends to push the vertebral bodies apart, and the tension provided by the ligaments which tends to pull the bodies together. Thus the vertebral segments and discs are firmly bound together by ligaments under tension: (1) a longitudinal system which binds all the vertebrae together into a mechanical unit (in other words, anterior and posterior longitudinal ligaments, supraspinous ligaments); (2) a longitudinal system which secures one segment to another (in other words interspinous, intertransverse and iliolumbar ligaments, and the ligamentum flavum). This arrangement accounts for the relative stability of the spine dissected free of musculature. Lucas (1970) noted the obvious similarity of the spine to a segmental column composed of alternating rigid and elastic elements. Such a column can be considered a modified elastic rod and so can be studied in the same manner as any flexible rod. Lucas propounded the hypothesis that the stability of the human ligamentous spine devoid of musculature can be predicted in the same terms as the stability of an equivalent elastic rod. Therefore the first phase of his study involved a review of the behaviour of elastic rods.

Consider an elastic rod clamped to a solid base at its bottom and subjected to a small vertical load at its top. If in addition to the vertical load a small lateral force is applied, a lateral displacement is produced. When the lateral force is removed the rod returns to its original position. This form of elastic equilibrium is called stable equilibrium. The vertical load may be increased, and with application and removal of the lateral force the same cycle of lateral displacement and elastic recovery can be repeated. When the vertical load reaches a certain magnitude, a very slight lateral force will produce a displacement which cannot be recovered by merely removing the lateral force. This condition is known as unstable equilibrium. A very slight further increase of the vertical load will cause a sudden lateral bending of the rod without additional lateral force. That phenomenon is called stability failure, or buckling. The vertical load at which failure occurs is called the critical load. The magnitude of the critical load can be expressed as $Pcr = C\pi^2/KL^2$ where

$$Pcr = \text{critical load}$$
$$C = \text{constant}$$
$$K = \text{rod flexibility}$$
$$L = \text{length of rod}$$

C depends on the shape of the buckling curve which in turn depends on the end-support conditions. The flexibility constant, K, represents the measure of the bending deformability of the rod and depends upon its material composition in addition to the size and shape of its cross-section.

Lucas and Bresler (1961) removed fresh adult spines at autopsy and studied the thoracic, lumbar and sacral regions. The spinal ligaments were preserved but the muscles were detached. Twelve spines were mounted in a

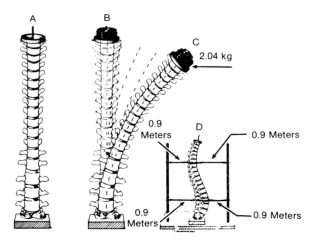

Figure 10.1   Adult thoracolumbar ligamentous spine, fixed at base and free at top, under vertical loading, and restrained at midthoracic and midlumbar levels in anteroposterior plane. A. before loading: B. during loading: C. stability failure occurring under 2.04 kg load: D. lateral view showing anteroposterior restraints (after Lucas and Bresler, 1961)

vertical position with the sacral portion securely fastened to a fixed base and loads were applied to the first thoracic vertebra. It appeared that the most flexible elements in the spines were located between the levels of the third and seventh thoracic vertebrae. The lumbosacral joint was found to be the least flexible of all (Figure **10.1**).

The effective flexibility of a spine is calculated by distributing the sum of the flexibilities for all elastic segments uniformly over the length of the spine. The effective flexibility (K) is equal to the sum of the flexibilities divided by the length of the spine. The critical load value for the spine may then be calculated by substituting the actual value established for K in the formula for critical load. For a representative spine the critical load value was calculated to be 2.09 kg (4.6 lb) – under such a vertical load the spine would be expected to buckle. The critical load value for the spine was determined independently by vertical loading. When fixed at the base and free at the top the spine failed at 1.95 kg (4.3 lb). Thus the thoracolumbar portion of the ligamentous adult spine does behave like an elastic rod and the mechanical factors which govern the behaviour of elastic rods can be applied to the human spine.

When upright the normal living person has adequate intrinsic and extrinsic support. It is obvious that the unconscious adult cannot remain upright because of lack of extrinsic support, since the weight of the torso far exceeds the critical load of 2 kg (4.4 lb) for the ligamentous spine. In the upright and conscious adult, with the spine fixed at top and bottom by muscles, the critical load value for the spine is approximately 33 kg (73 lb), which is close to the average combined weight of the torso, head and upper extremities. This implies a close relationship between weight of the trunk and critical load value in an individual standing relaxed.

In considering the mechanical factors which govern the behaviour of elastic rods, there are three variables which affect spine stability and deformities: the length, the end-support conditions and the flexibility. The critical load value varies inversely with the square of the length. The longer the spine, the more limber it becomes and the greater is its tendency to buckle and deform under vertical loading. The end-support conditions of the spine restrain it and add to its stability. The flexibility of the spine depends on its material characteristics and the shape of its discs, as well as on restraints offered by the interspinal ligaments. Morris, Lucas, and Bresler (1961) showed that the flexibility between two vertebrae varies directly with the square of the vertical height of the disc and indirectly with the square of the horizontal diameter of the body. Thus for a given load and cross-section an increase in the height of the disc and the length of the ligaments tends to increase the apparent flexibility, while an increase in the cross-sectional size of the disc tends to reduce apparent flexibility. Because of the proportionally greater height of the lumbar disc, the range of intervertebral motion is somewhat greater in the lumbar region; but because of the greater horizontal diameter, the flexibility is less than in the thoracic region. Lucas (1970) believes that idiopathic scoliosis is due to a stability failure of the spine induced by increased elasticity of the intervertebral structures at a time when the extrinsic support of the spine is inadequate. In this condition the spine behaves according to the laws governing elastic rods. It appears to be a familial disease primarily affecting adolescent girls.

In the previous chapter it was noted that various workers have shown that on vertical compression of spinal segments the vertebral end-plates are the first structures to fracture. Study of autopsy material and living patients has shown that the compressive strength of the vertebral bodies on static loading is between 200 and 1200 kg (440 and 2640 lb), the differences being dependent on the age and sex of the individual (Perey, 1957). To a certain extent the vertebrae exhibit elasticity. The mean compression before fracturing of the vertebral body is about 15 per cent (Nachemson, 1962). Ruff (1945) also calculated what part of the total body weight is supported by different vertebral bodies (Table 10.1).

Table 10.1   Fracture load of selected vertebral bodies and the percentage of the total body weight which those vertebral bodies support (from Ruff, 1945)

Vertebra	Fracture load in kg	Load carried by each vertebra as per cent of total body weight
C4	275	7
T1	450	20
T4	600	25
L1	900	50
L5	1000	60

Other axial compression tests carried out by Messerer (1880), Lange (1902), Ellis (1944), and more recently by Roaf (1960) and Farfan (1973) generally agree with these results. Investigation of spinal fractures occurring in catapult-ejected pilots has given reliable figures for the forces necessary to fracture their vertebrae. In 23 ejections from one aircraft at a maximum acceleration of 15–20 g, no fractures occurred; in 29 escapes from another type of aircraft at maximum acceleration 20–25 g, 12 pilots fractured their spines (Hirsch and Nachemson, 1961; Laurell and Nachemson, 1961). Thus all vertebral fractures occurred when the spine was subjected to forces around 1000 kg (2200 lb). In static loading experiments the stress tolerance of the intervertebral discs has been measured using an intervertebral disc with adjacent slices of bone under compression in various types of apparatus. The reports of several authors are compared in Table 10.2.

In a more recent review Morris (1973) states that compression tests have shown that the disc behaves as an elastic body only up to a maximum total pressure of 635 kg (1400 lb) (in specimens from young adults). In specimens

Table 10.2   Fracture loads for lumbar spine specimens (from Nachemson, (1962)

Author	Preparation	Number of specimens tested	Fracture load mean value (kg)
Bartelink (1957)	One disc and parts of adjacent vertebrae	10	320
Evans (1957)	One disc and parts of adjacent vertebrae	96	390
Perey (1957)	One disc and parts of adjacent vertebrae	40	560
Brown-Hansen-Yorra (1957)	One disc and parts of adjacent vertebrae	5	550
Decoulx-Rieunau (1958)	Two discs and three adjacent vertebrae	9	700
Evans-Lissner (1959)	Pelvis and five lumbar vertebrae with discs { 7 embalmed / 3 fresh		400 / 250

from older persons, the elastic limit is approximately 158.8 kg (350 lb). Beyond this amount, the disc is rapidly deformed by very little additional pressure. Compression forces have been imposed up to the point of failure of a particular segment of the spine under study. This failure is characterized by an audible crack followed by leakage of sanguinous fluid from one of the vertebrae (usually the superior), through the vascular foramen, and occasionally at some point along the attachment of the peripheral fibres of the annulus to the vertebral bodies. The evidence of failure is often difficult to visualize either upon gross examination or radiographically. It may consist of compression of a few spicules of bone, cracks in the end-plate, or collapse of the plate. It has been shown that this failure occurs in specimens from young persons at a compressive load of 453.6 kg to 771.1 kg (1000 to 1700 lb). When specimens from older persons were studied, the critical load was much less, even as little as 136.1 kg (300 lb).

When a subject stands upright with a heavy weight held in the arms stretched out in front of the trunk, a large force is generated at the lumbo-sacral junction resulting from the very short lever arm from which the erectores spinae muscles are obliged to act. The ratio of the anterior to the posterior lever arm is approximately 10:1 so when a weight of 100 kg (220 lb) is held, there is a reaction of 1100 kg (2424 lb) on the lumbosacral junction (Figure **10.2**).

As forces of 1000 kg (2200 lb) or so cannot be tolerated by the vertebral tissues we must question how the spine can support these apparent loads to which it is subjected. The spine is attached to the sides of, and within, two chambers, the thoracic and abdominal cavities, which are separated by a diaphragm. The thoracic cavity is filled largely with air and the abdominal

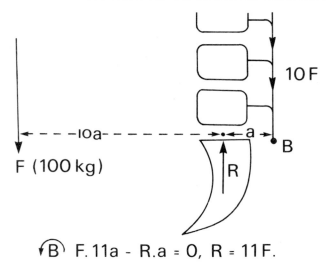

√B̄ F. 11a - R.a = 0, R = 11F.

Figure 10.2 Weight (F) of 100 kg held at arms' length produces a reaction of 1100 kg on the lumbosacral junction

cavity with a semiliquid mass. It was postulated that the action of the trunk muscles converts these chambers into nearly rigid walled cylinders, both of which are capable of resisting a part of the force generated by loading the trunk and thereby relieve the load on the spine itself.

Morris, Lucas, and Bresler (1961) studied this hypothesis and they showed that, during the act of lifting, the action of the intercostal muscles and the muscles of the shoulder girdle rendered the thoracic cage quite rigid. An increase in intrathoracic pressure resulted, converting the thoracic cage and the spine into a sturdy unit capable of transmitting large forces. By contraction of the diaphragm and the muscles of the abdominal wall, the abdominal contents were compressed into a semirigid mass, thereby making the abdominal cavity a semirigid cylinder. The force of weight lifted by the arms is thus transmitted to the spinal column by the muscles of the shoulder girdle, principally the trapezius, and then on to the abdominal cylinder and the pelvis, partly through the spinal column and partly through the rigid rib cage and abdomen. The larger the weight lifted, the greater the activity of the trunk, chest and abdominal musculature was found to be. Also, a concomitant increase in intracavitary pressures resulted. Considering the effects of the increased cavitary pressures, the calculated force on the lumbosacral disc during lifting of any load was found to be decreased by 30 per cent and the load on the lower thoracic portion of the spine was about 50 per cent less than it would have been without support by the trunk. Thus, when 100 kg (220 lb) are lifted, instead of approximately 1100 kg (2424 lb) of force being transmitted along the spine, only about 600 kg (1320 lb) is actually transmitted.

Bartelink (1957) described the role of the abdominal pressure in relieving the pressure on the lumbar intervertebral discs. He measured the intra-abdominal pressure with a balloon in the stomach of subjects lifting weights and bending over to different degrees. In extreme flexion of the trunk the pressure is not so high as when the hands are 25–40 cm away from the floor, in which position the pressure is greatest. If the lifter continues slowly to straighten out, the pressure drops rather rapidly and is already low with the body still bent over 15–20°. In the upright position, whatever the load in the hands, the pressure is usually very low and never significant. In Bartelink's experiments the equipment to measure the sudden high elevations of pressure was not available, which was unfortunate because he believed that the reflex contraction of the abdominal wall muscles lasted only a very short time. Eie and Wehn (1962) measured pressures in the abdomen and thorax simultaneously by means of one balloon-catheter in the stomach and one in the oesophagus. They found the pressure in the stomach to be always positive and to fluctuate with respiration. The pressure rose with forward bending and reached its maximum at about 45° of forward bending. The pressure in the thorax was always lower than the pressure in the abdomen. The highest intra-abdominal pressure recorded by a weightlifter was 225 mmHg, while a less muscular man did not succeed in producing more than 125 mmHg. All these observations make it clear that there is a relationship between lifting and intra-abdominal pressure. Bartelink postulated that some of the load of the upper trunk is transmitted, via the somatic cavity, down to the pelvis by this 'muscular skeleton' (Figure **10.3**).

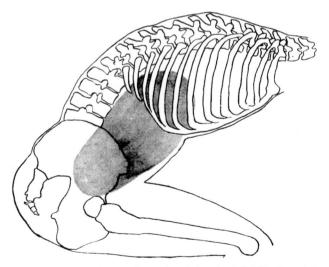

Figure 10.3   Diagram to suggest how the abdominal fluid ball, as it is attached to the costal margin, would provide some support for the upper trunk, in case of lifting with the trunk flexed forward (from Bartelink, 1957)

With electromyographic studies of the abdominal wall during weight-lifting Bartelink found that the rectus abdominis muscles, which are mainly concerned in longitudinal pull, do not contract. The electromyographs suggested that perhaps the main action responsible for raising the intra-abdominal pressure is supplied by the transverse abdominal muscles which do not have a significant vertical component. The absence of action of the abdominal recti during weightlifting fits in with what Floyd and Silver (1950) found for the behaviour of the abdominal wall during straining: that there is no action of the recti.

Stillwell (1973) describes this phenomenon as a clinical application of the Law of Laplace which describes the relationship between the transmural pressure, the tension in the wall of a container at any point and the amount of curvature of the wall at that point. The intra-abdominal cavity is irregularly shaped. In the coronal plane it is elliptical except at the top where the two leaves of the diaphragm have individual curvatures. In the sagittal plane it is essentially elliptical with a smaller radius of curvature at the upper pole than in the anterior wall. In the transverse plane the anterior and lateral walls of the cavity are elliptical. The posterior wall is unchanging and need not be considered herein, and the inferior pole is relatively unyielding and has a small radius of curvature in all planes (Figure **10.4**).

Stillwell continues:

When the individual takes a deep breath and holds it, the diaphragmatic leaves are flattened somewhat. This reaction is associated with an increase in their radii of curvature both in the coronal and sagittal planes but still the two-leaf structure makes it a more efficient producer of pressure than it would be if it formed a single (flatter) curve. The forward displacement of the anterior abdominal wall by the abdominal contents decreases the radii of curvature of this region in both the transverse and sagittal planes, thus enabling it to exert more pressure for each unit of tension. In the actual situation the gaseous abdominal contents are compressible so that there will be some reduction in the volume of the 'fluid ball' rather than the theoretically isovolumic change in its shape. The protrusion of the abdomen also will permit the transverse and oblique muscles to perform their isometric contraction at a more advantageous length from the point of view of developing tension.

Tightening up the abdominal wall without preliminary inspiration may lead to flattening of the wall and decreased ability to compress the contents both from the viewpoint of the Law of Laplace and from the length–tension relationship. From the viewpoint of the Law of Laplace the abdominal wall should also be less effective in the 'long waisted' person.

The patient who has an increased volume of abdominal contents, whether it be fat, a well advanced pregnancy, or a tumour, may have to develop more than the normal amount of tension in the abdominal wall in order to exert the requisite pressure on the contents to help to 'unload' the lumbar spine. In the obese person, the abdominal muscles also may be in poor condition from prolonged disuse. The likelihood that they can be strengthened sufficiently to do the job will be enhanced if the demands of the job can be diminished by reducing the intra-abdominal fat.

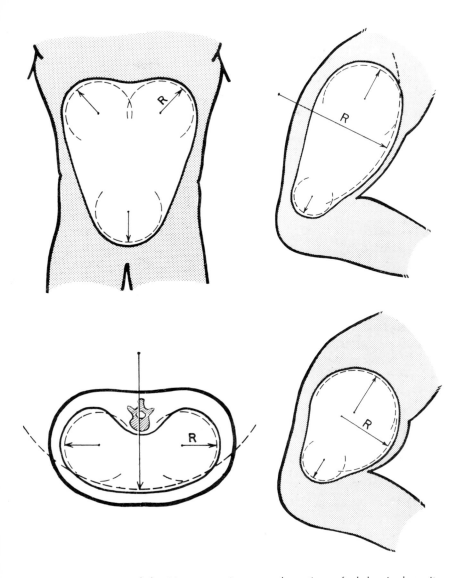

Figure 10.4 Upper left. Diagrammatic coronal section of abdominal cavity showing radii of curvature of its upper and lower boundaries. Each arrow represents a radius (R) though only one is labelled. Upper right. Diagrammatic sagittal section of abdominal cavity showing radii of curvature of upper, lower and anterior boundaries. Lower left. Diagrammatic transverse section of abdominal cavity showing radii of curvature of anterior and lateral boundaries. Lower right. Diagrammatic representation of changes in radii of curvature during Valsalva manoeuver. (see Upper Right) (from Stillwell, 1973)

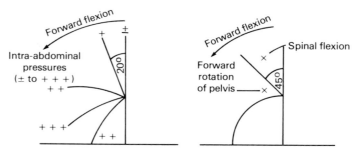

Figure 10.5   Comparison of intra-abdominal pressures and skeletal mechanics during trunk forward flexion

Bartelink (1957) reminds us that the transverse abdominal muscle anatomically belongs to the same group as the diaphragm and the transverse thoracic muscle. These muscles surround the upper part of the fluid ball and by their contraction create the muscular skeleton much in the same way as invertebrates are able to create a support that enables them to drive forward the front end of their bodies. The abdominal fluid ball according to this reasoning would be genetically very old, and part of the reflex might even be an inborn reflex. Animals in general undoubtedly make an extensive use of the protection of their spines by the tensed somatic cavity. The position of the lungs outside the fluid ball enables breathing to go on when the abdomen is used for support and cannot be relaxed. This means that the range of flight of an animal having the lungs outside the fluid ball is greater than that of an animal who has its lungs in the single body cavity, which can just make a spurt and then has to stop to breathe.

Farfan (1978) has argued that the human lumbar spine, although commonly abused, is highly advanced along the evolutionary scale. The adaptation of man's spine and hip is not an incompletely developed physical structure but a vastly superior muscle–ligament system to that of other primates for lifting weights. When man bends forward to touch hands to toes, motion occurs in the lumbar spine as well as at the hips. Most of the spinal flexion occurs by the time the trunk is inclined 45° forward. The remainder of the arc of motion is brought about by forward rotation of the pelvis. We can compare this sequence to Bartelink's (1957) intra-abdominal pressures in weightlifters (Figure **10.5**).

In the first stage of forward flexion the lumbar joints flex as the back extensors lower the body weight. At a point near 45° of forward flexion the posterior ligamentous system, which has been developing tension gradually, rapidly tightens thereby relieving the strain on the back muscles. Further forward flexion then occurs with pelvic rotation under control of the hip extensors, allowing the trunk above the fully flexed hip joint to be brought to a horizontal position. In straightening up, the rhythm is reversed with the pelvis first moving backward followed by lumbar spine extension.

Because he has a greater number of free lumbar joints and a greater thickness of lumbar discs, man has the greatest degree of lumbar spine flexibility of all the primates. Farfan questions why the lumbar spine of man should be so flexible when in normal design one might expect the main supporting beam to be a rigid member like that of a crane instead of a flexible rod. Perhaps the answer lies in the fact that the configuration of man's spine did not evolve for the purpose of proficient weightlifting. We have already seen the flexibility put to good use in a locomotor role. Another indication that the prime function of the trunk musculature is not to raise external loads is the abundance of the trunk muscles. Farfan has calculated that the available power exceeds that necessary for lifting. He suggests that the extra extensor power of the spine is there to permit accelerated motions of the spine.

Because there is a marked lumbosacral angle in man and the spinous processes of the fourth and fifth lumbar vertebrae and of the first and second sacral segments are small, the supraspinous ligament passes some distance behind the vertebral processes. The ligamentous sheet, however, remains attached to the tips of these processes by ligamentous extensions. This 'lordotic' arrangement provides two advantages: (1) as the ligament is behind the tips of the spinous processes, its leverage is greatly increased; and (2) when the ligament is stretched it pulls back the fourth and fifth lumbar vertebrae, thus reducing the forward shearing force produced by the weight lifted. In other anthropoids the posterior ligamentous system runs a slightly curved course continuous with the thoracic curve and is therefore unable to neutralize shear loads (Figure **10.6**).

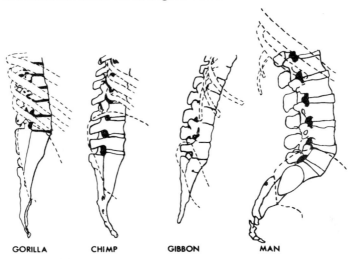

GORILLA   CHIMP   GIBBON   MAN

Figure 10.6   Lateral view of articulated primate skeletons – gorilla, chimp, gibbon and man (from Farfan, 1978)

Because in man there is a permanent lordosis, Farfan describes the lower lumbar joints as always subjected to a shearing force even in the relaxed upright stance. For this reason the apophyseal joints of the lower two or three segments have developed a reorientation which supports this shear when the posterior ligamentous system is relaxed. The overall mechanical advantage of the anatomical arrangements in man leave him with an over-abundance of power to attain the upright posture and to allow accelerated actions of the trunk and upper extremities. It is difficult to understand in the evolutionary scheme how hand—eye coordination could have evolved in the absence of these powerful erector mechanisms (Farfan, 1978).

IN SUMMARY

65. The spinal column possesses intrinsic stability due to the binding together of the vertebral segments and discs by ligaments under tension. This arrangement accounts for the relative stability of the spine dissected free of musculature as it behaves like a modified elastic rod. In addition the spine has extrinsic stability provided by the muscle support.

66. Compression tests on vertebral bodies have shown that failure occurs at loads of the order of 500–800 kg (1100–1760 lb) in specimens from young persons. Investigations of injuries sustained by catapult ejections of jet pilots showed that vertebral compression fractures occurred at forces just over 20 g. Yet when the subject lifts a weight of 100 kg (220 lb) the lumbosacral junction is subjected to a reaction greater than 1000 kg (2200 lb). How can the vertebral tissues tolerate these loads?

67. It does so by converting the thoracic and abdominal cavities into semirigid walled cylinders of air and semisolids respectively, which are capable of transmitting large forces and operate with a much greater lever arm than that of the erectores spinae muscles. The calculated force on the lumbosacral disc during lifting is found to be reduced by 30 per cent when using this 'muscular skeleton'.

68. Electromyographs show that the increase in intra-abdominal pressure needed to convert the somatic cavity into this fluid ball is brought about by contraction of the transverse abdominal muscle, which anatomically belongs to the same group as the diaphragm and the transverse thoracic muscle. Is this therefore a genetically very old mechanism? Certainly animals in general make an extensive use of tensed somatic cavities to protect their spines.

69. Farfan has shown that the human spine is highly advanced along the evolutionary scale. The adaptation of man's spine and hip is a vastly superior muscle—ligament system than that of other primates for weightlifting.

11 The biomechanics of backache

The posterior elements are composed of the apophyseal or facet joints, the intertransverse ligaments, the ligamenta flava, the inferior half of the laminae and the spinous process (Figure **11.1**). Their role in the mechanics of the spine is usually determined from observations of the motion of fresh autopsy specimens before and after ablation of the posterior elements.

Markolf (1972) performed static loading tests on fresh human spinal segments to measure the deformation of the thoracic and lumbar joints in response to forces applied in various directions. He found that the articular processes and related ligaments contributed to the mechanical rigidity of the intervertebral joint during bending and torsion. These processes are of particular mechanical significance in the extension stiffness of the thoracic and lumbar joints and in torsional stiffness of the lumbar joints. The torsional stiffness showed a marked change at the eleventh and twelfth thoracic

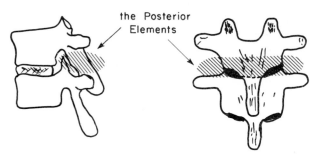

the Posterior
Elements

Figure 11.1 A diagrammatic representation of how the posterior elements were ablated by cutting through the darkened area. The dotted line in the posterior view of the motion segment indicates the location of the yellow ligament. (after White and Hirsch, 1971)

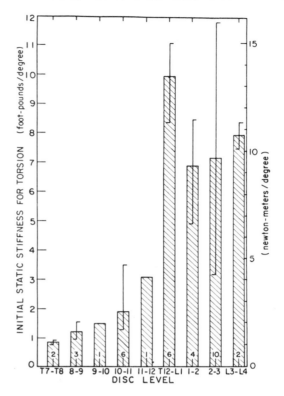

Figure 11.2   The static rotatory stiffness for torsion changes abruptly between the tenth thoracic and the first lumbar vertebrae. (from Markolf, 1972)

vertebrae with marked stiffness below that level and relatively little stiffness higher in the column (Figure **11.2**).

For his axial tension and compression tests, Markolf used vertebra–disc–vertebra specimens with the posterior structures removed as he referred to previous compression studies by Hirsch and Nachemson (1954), which had verified that the articular processes and ligaments are not important for the transmission of axial loads through the spinal column. Similarly, preliminary tests revealed that the posterior structures had no measurable influence upon the shear displacements of an intervertebral joint when the forces were applied in an anterior-to-posterior or medial-to-lateral direction. The curves for lateral bending were essentially the same before and after removal of the posterior elements (Figure **11.3**), as were the curves for flexion (Figure **11.4**).

The extension curves indicate that removal of the posterior structures substantially reduced the stiffness of both the thoracic and the lumbar interspaces (Figure **11.5**). For torsion the before and after curves differed little for

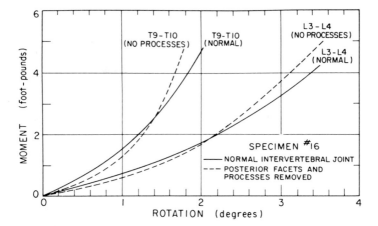

Figure 11.3 Effect of the articular processes and posterior elements on the moment–rotation behaviour of a thoracic and a lumbar intervertebral joint. (1 foot-pound force = 1.356 newton-meters) In lateral bending (from Markolf, 1972)

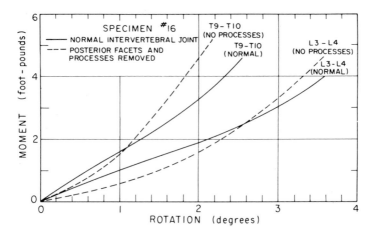

Figure 11.4 Effect of the articular processes and posterior elements on the moment–rotation behaviour of a thoracic and a lumbar intervertebral joint. (1 foot-pound force = 1.356 newton-meters) In flexion (from Markolf, 1972)

the thoracic interspace but were markedly different for the lumbar joint (Figure **11.6**).

These similarities and differences were expected by Markolf. During lateral bending most of the posterior ligaments are not stretched and there is little impingement of the articular processes. During flexion the posterior ligaments are put on a stretch and during extension impingement of the articular processes, one against the other, must increase bending resistance.

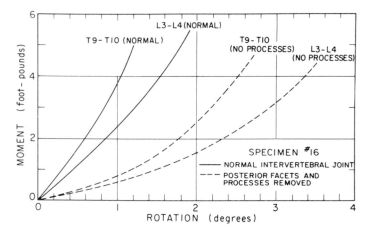

Figure 11.5   Effect of the articular processes and posterior elements on the moment–rotation behaviour of a thoracic and a lumbar intervertebral joint. (1 foot-pound force = 1.356 newton-meters) In extension (from Markolf, 1972)

The effect on the limitation of torsion by the posterior elements of the lumbar vertebrae alone is consistent with Davis's (1959) observations, as described in Chapter 7, on the medial inclination of the thoracic inter-vertebral articular facets. These indicated that simple rotation can occur in the mid-thoracic region but elsewhere in the thoracic spine rotation must be accompanied by lateral shearing.

White and Hirsch (1971) examined the significance of the posterior elements in the mechanics of the thoracic spine. They, like Markolf, found that after removal of the posterior elements there was more extension for a given force but in addition they noted a larger amount of flexion and greater axial rotation. Direct observation confirmed that the spinous processes and the facets limited extension and the findings supported Akerblom's (1948) suggestion that the ligamentum flavum limits forward flexion. The tests paradoxically supported the contention that in the thoracic spine the align-ment of the facets is such that axial rotation is a relatively free motion. This resulted from the elastic nature of the observed restriction of the axial rotation prior to the removal of the posterior elements. This suggested that the ligamentum flavum resisted this rotation. The resistance was not that of rigid, abrupt blocking that would be expected with bony resistance, but rather that of an increasing elastic resistance.

Jamiolkowska (1973) studied the planes and axes of rotation of the vertebral column from $C_2/_3$ to L_5/S_1 by photographing the vertebrae from three directions. She confirmed that the rotation axes do not pass through the nucleus pulposus. In the lumbar region the rotation axes pass behind the vertebral canal, and in the thoracic and cervical segments they pass in front of the vertebral column. The backward displacement of the axis was greatest

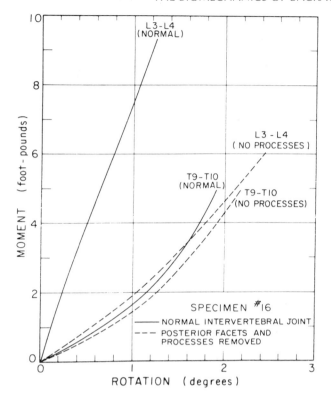

Figure 11.6 Effect of the articular processes and posterior elements on the moment–rotation behaviour of a thoracic and a lumbar intervertebral joint. (1 foot-pound force = 1.356 newton-meters) In torsion (from Markolf, 1972)

in the L_5/S_1 segment, extending to the end of the spinous process of L_5. The greatest forward displacement was in segments C_7/T_1 and $T_1/_2$. The position of all the axes was not in the same straight line. The planes of rotation of the motion segments have different angles of inclination to the horizontal. In the $T_{11}/_{12}$ segment there is a sudden forward shift of the axes. The axes of the next thoracic segments up to $T_3/_4$ are situated in almost a single vertical line in front of the bodies (Figure **11.7**).

The studies on vertebrae show up two important findings. Firstly the difference between the thoracic and lumbar portions of the spine, and secondly the abrupt nature of the change from one to the other in the thoracolumbar junction. The anatomical studies are consistent with the *in vivo* studies of Gregersen and Lucas (1967) in all parts of the thoracolumbar spine. As the torsional stiffness showed a marked change at T_{11} and T_{12}, Markolf (1972) hypothesized that this discontinuity represents a site of structural weakness for torsional stresses to the spinal column.

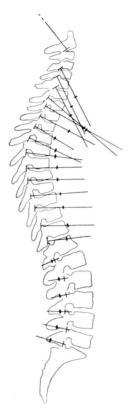

Figure 11.7   Scheme of the vertebral column showing the position of the planes and axes of rotation of different segments (from Jamiolkowska, 1973)

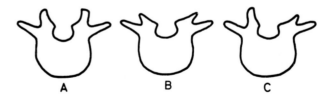

Figure 11.8   A : B : C   Three types of orientation of the facets in the lumbar spine (after Maslow and Rothman, 1975)

Maslow and Rothman (1975) described the inclinations of the articulating surfaces of the facets as 45° to the sagittal plane at the $L_1/_2$ level as in A (Figure **11.8**). The inclinations assume an increasingly frontal orientation moving caudally as represented by the L_5/S_1 level in B. There is an asymmetry of orientation, as in C, in the facets of 20 per cent of lower lumbar spines.

The more obliquely orientated a facet is, the less it can resist rotary stress. In an asymmetric situation, when one facet is oblique, rotation occurs toward that side. Farfan and Sullivan (1967) suggested that abnormal stress is placed on the posterolateral disc by such asymmetry; they found a high correlation between asymmetrical orientation of the facet joints and the level of disc pathology. Furthermore, the same high correlation was seen between the side of the disc prolapse and the side of the more obliquely orientated facet.

We may have discovered already many of the clues which point to (at least some of) the predisposing causes of mechanical derangements of the human thoracolumbar spine. During walking the spine undergoes axial rotation in opposite directions above and below a transition point at the level of T_6 to T_8 (Gregersen and Lucas, 1967). Anatomical studies show that rotation occurs easily in this region but elsewhere (especially in the lumbar region) axial rotation must be accompanied by lateral shearing (Davis, 1959; Gregersen and Lucas, 1967). Farfan et al. (1970) showed that axial rotation in the lumbar region was capable of producing damage to the intervertebral joint, and disc rupture induced by torsion produced changes similar to those seen in naturally occurring disc degeneration. The posterior elements of the

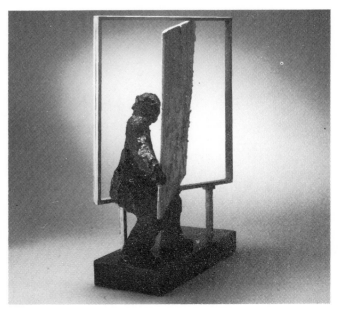

Figure 11.9 Carrying large objects extends and locks the thoracic spine; thus subsequent rotation must take place in the lumbar spine, a region normally allowing flexion and extension but limiting rotation

thoracic and lumbar vertebrae limit extension (White and Hirsch, 1971; Markolf, 1972); conversely extension of the thoracic spine will lock the vertebrae together thus preventing subsequent rotation. Hence if the thoracic spine is extended and locked, for example by carrying a large object, subsequent rotation cannot take place in this region and if rotation has to take place it must do so in the lumbar region (Figure **11.9**).

This will produce disc rupture in the lumbar region especially at the level L_5/S_1 where the axis of rotation is displaced backwards the farthest (Jamiolkowska, 1973). This explains the frequency of 'back injury' associated, not so much by lifting heavy items, but by attempting to lift and twist with awkward loads so that extension and rotary movements are involved together.

Carrying small weights in the hands shifts the transition point higher in the spine towards the cervicothoracic junction (Gregersen and Lucas, 1967). Repeated rotation at this level will produce continuous shearing forces especially at the C_7/T_1 level where the greatest forward displacement of the axis of rotation exists (Jamiolkowska). Thus continual carrying of small loads, for example shopping baskets, may lead to facet wear and tear and lower cervical disc disease often with brachialgia.

We adopt several mechanisms to lessen the effect of rotary moments. These moments are smaller the nearer an object is carried to the axis of rotation. This may explain the different carrying habits of men and women

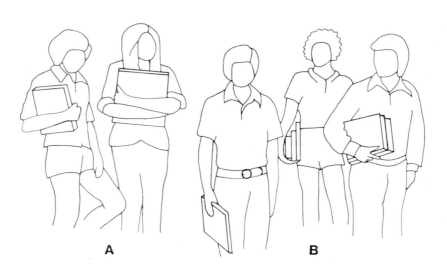

A   **B**

Figure 11.10 Methods of carrying books. (A) in all type I carrying methods, the short edges of the book rest on the hip or in front of the body. (B) In type II methods, the books are either pinched from above or supported from below by the hand or the hand and arm. (from Jenni and Jenni, 1976)

as described by Jenni and Jenni (1976). They noticed that females tend to clasp books against their chests while males carry them at their sides (Figure **11.10**). This can be explained by the ratios of hip width to shoulder width which are different for males and females, so both sexes carry in a way such that their burden is as near to the axis of rotation as possible, males carrying books close to their narrow hips, and females close to their narrow chests. In India, heavy objects are carried on the head and the graceful posture of many head-carriers is well known. Here the load could not be nearer to the axis of rotation. Roaf (1977) reminds us that throughout history a bent figure carrying a heavy load has been used to depict the impoverished, down-trodden 'have-nots' of this world, traditionally suggesting, unhappiness, fatigue and dejection. There is, however, some evidence that people who walk and run and move but do not carry very heavy loads preserve better postures throughout their lives – drovers, nomads, camel-drivers and so on are famed for their striking upright postures which suggest happiness.

Davis (1968) tells us that the divorce of the upper limb from locomotor function resulting from bipedalism not only promoted manual dexterity but also permitted adoption of a habit of moving things from place to place. The killing of wild ungulates at a distance from home necessitated and promoted the selection of transporting abilities, either the male having to carry the food to the mother or the mother having to carry the helpless infant to the food, or both. This hypothesis is attractive and suggests that the carrying of burdens in the hands is a longstanding feature of human ancestry. When one examines the magnitudes and frequency of transport of burdens, one realizes that it is only in very recent times that man has handled heavy objects with great frequency. A carnivorous diet is a concentrated and compact form of food, so that quite small and infrequent burdens would serve the dietary needs of an early human family. Today's 5-year-old child only weighs about 20 kg (44 lb) and can walk considerable distances long before this. Thus it is not improbable that, up to the beginnings of modern materialistic civilization, burdens in excess of an infant's weight were not transported with any frequency. It is only in the past 5000 or 10 000 years that frequent heavy load-bearing has become part of the human pattern of behaviour. Although nowadays few industrial workers and housewives are persistently required to undertake heavy manual labour, there are many occasions when they have to lift and carry burdens far in excess of 20 kg (44 lb).

Wood (1976) believes this to be too simplistic a concept, largely because increased lifting stress would appear to apply to all of us, whereas back pain is by no means universal. A minority are affected in early maturity, and in these people the search for precipitating factors may well be most profitable. Against a background of spinal structures stressed by the physical demands of our way of life, one would expect variation in the ability to withstand these forces; the vulnerable could well be those whose supporting system has less reserve with which to adapt to these stresses. Alternatively, Wood says it may be occurrences like an exceptional twisting or rotational stress that are responsible, out of relation to the diffuse increase in forces for which physical evolution has not fitted us.

IN SUMMARY

70.   The posterior elements of the vertebrae are of particular mechanical significance in the extension stiffness of the thoracic and lumbar joints and in the torsional stiffness of the lumbar joints.

71.   Many of the conclusions described earlier in this monograph have been recalled to present examples of the way in which mechanical factors may affect disc degeneration.

72.   Explanations are offered for disc degeneration at the lumbosacral junction following awkward lifting, and disc degeneration at the cervicothoracic junction following repetitive carrying.

73.   Methods of carrying are given as examples of the ways in which mankind reduces the risks involved. Davis (1968) hypothesizes that the problem of prolapsed discs is associated with frequent heavy load-bearing.

Part 2
The Abnormal Back

12 Spinal stenosis

Rather than incriminating increased lifting stress as the universal cause of back pain, Wood (1976) proposed a search for precipitating factors in that minority of persons affected in early maturity. One anatomical variation which has been shown to predispose to low back pain with leg symptoms is lumbar canal stenosis or 'spinal stenosis'. Apart from its mechanical functions described in the previous chapters, the lumbar portion of the spine transmits the dural sac, lumbar and sacral nerve roots within a protected spinal canal. The bony canal is bounded anteriorly by the backs of the vertebral bodies and the intervertebral discs, and posterolaterally by the pedicles, articular facets and laminae. The dimensions of the bony canal are reduced by the posterior longitudinal ligament lying on the posterior aspect of the vertebral bodies and posterolaterally by the ligamentum flavum (see Figure **6.1**). The size of the vertebral canal varies between individual spines and among segments of the same spine. At the first lumbar level the canal is normally oval and this cross-sectional shape is nearly always present at the second lumbar levels (Figure **12.1**). At the third level more canals are triangular or deltoid with the articular facets indenting the canal to form lateral recesses. At the last lumbar levels the triangular and deltoid shapes predominate. The shallow lateral recesses are occupied almost entirely by the nerve roots with the result that any further intrusion into this space will affect their mobility and produce nerve root damage (Jayson and Nelson, 1979). It is the deltoid or trefoil canal which is found in association with spinal stenosis.

Lumbar canal stenosis results from a variable degree of spondylosis super-imposed on variable developmental narrowing which combine to produce critical cauda equina compression and the typical clinical syndrome (Roberts, 1978).

149

POSTERIOR

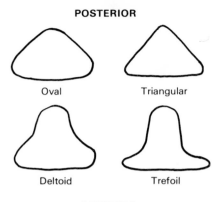

ANTERIOR

Figure 12.1   Spinal canal shapes (from Jayson and Nelson, 1979)

Developmental stenosis occurs as congenital narrowing of the sagittal or coronal spinal diameters. The pedicles are shorter and the posterior joints are closer to the midline than normal creating prominent posterolateral impressions on the cross-sectional appearance of the canal. A similar configuration is seen in achondroplasia. Acquired stenosis can result from several causes including chronic disc degeneration with posterior joint osteoarthritis. Often a combined developmental and acquired stenosis is seen and symptoms occur for the first time in patients of 40–50 years of age because of degenerative encroachments upon the developmentally shallow canal. In the presence of lumbar spondylosis the lumina of the spinal canal and the exit canals of the spinal nerves are reduced anteriorly by the bulging annulus fibrosus of the discs and by osteophytes along the posterior margins of the vertebral bodies, and posteriorly by degenerative changes around the posterior intervertebral joints. Thickening of the ligamenta flava can also reduce the canal's dimensions and further concertina-like folding of an already thickened ligamentum flavum by spinal extension results in still more pressure on the posterior aspect of the theca. Full extension has also been shown to narrow the exit canals and foramina in normal non-stenotic spines. Thus the dimensions of the vertebral canal are not constant but are affected by posture and movement. Not only does extension of the spine decrease the cross-sectional area of the canal and the size of the inter-vertebral foramina but spinal flexion increases the size of these apertures.

The patient is usually a middle-aged man with a long history of low back pain which appears to be related to activity and relieved by rest. The back pain and subsequent root pains are non-specific except that the latter are rarely aggravated by coughing and sneezing, presumably because the contents of the lumbar canal are so constricted that they cannot be displaced further (Brish, Lerner, and Braham, 1964). The patient then notices numbness, tingling and sometimes muscle weakness in one or both lower limbs which comes on with walking and is relieved by rest.

A typical patient would be symptom-free at rest but on walking might develop pain and paraesthesiae starting in the thigh or calf and spreading throughout the limb. The walking distance gradually becomes reduced and eventually he may be able to walk only 50–100 m before he is brought to rest. Unlike vascular intermittent claudication, the patients are often able to walk on with difficulty. Sitting or crouching bring relief within 15–30 min because these positions flex the spine. A small group of patients only have unilateral symptoms.

Careful examination usually reveals a slightly stiff back, a minimal reduction of straight leg raising and the ankle jerk may be absent on one or both sides. Exercising the patient often provokes symptoms and is a useful confirmatory procedure. At this stage the symptoms are usually relieved by flexion and aggravated by extension of the spine. Unlike patients with vascular claudication who find standing helpful, those with neurogenic claudication find that standing aggravates the discomfort. Patients in the neurogenic group take longer to recover after rest. Although there is a fair degree of overlap between the two groups, Hawkes and Roberts (1980) stated that an individual taking more than 30 min to recover is very likely to have neurogenic claudication.

The diagnosis is made radiographically and can often be suspected from measurements made on plain radiographs. Myelography and lumbar radiculography, epidurography, ascending lumbar venography, computed tomography and ultrasonographic scanning are well reviewed by Hawkes and Roberts.

The natural history is of insidious deterioration but a lumbar corset which maintains the spine in a slightly flexed position might help. Otherwise activities should be reduced and instruction given on posture. Further treatment is surgical decompression.

IN SUMMARY

74. The spinal canal in cross-section is normally oval in the upper lumbar region and triangular or trefoil in the lower lumbar region. If it is trefoil throughout the lumbar spine the cauda equina and the spinal nerve roots, which occupy the lateral recesses, are restricted. This condition is known as lumbar canal stenosis or spinal stenosis.

75. Further encroachment into the canal can result from a thickened ligamentum flavum, particularly when it is buckled by extension of the lumbar spine.

76. Spinal stenosis can be developmental, acquired (by disc degeneration or posterior joint osteoarthritis) or both. When the cause is

acquired superimposed on congenital, symptoms start in the 40–50 year decade. It occurs three times as often in males.

77.   Symptoms are of neurogenic claudication. Non-specific low back pain and root pains are followed by paraesthesiae in the lower limbs which come on with walking and are relieved by rest. Sitting or crouching bring relief because these positions flex the spine. Standing, and particularly standing with the lumbar spine in extension, aggravate the condition.

78.   The diagnosis is confirmed radiographically. Treatment is a lumbar corset which maintains the spine in slight flexion or surgical decompression.

13 Prolapsed intervertebral disc

Chapter 11 described one of the mechanisms of classical prolapse of the lumbar intervertebral disc. Although nearly all authors agree that in Britain two people in every hundred visit their medical practitioner every year complaining of low back pain, there is little agreement as to how much of this back pain can be attributed to the intervertebral disc. On the one hand Cyriax (1969) ascribes over 90 per cent of all organic symptoms of the lower back to disc disease whereas Dixon (1976) believes prolapsed intervertebral disc to be the most overdiagnosed cause of back pain, and Wyke (1976) emphasizes that less than 5 per cent of patients with backache have prolapsed discs. Many authors simply write that disc disease is common and refer to the 15 per cent or so incidence of pathological discs seen in routine post-mortems. Williams (1974) states that the disc between L_5 and S_1 has ruptured in the majority of all persons by the age of 20 years and, as a result, most people at this age are subject to pain even though they have not yet experienced any significant discomfort. They do not have long to wait because setting aside Adams's (1971) quoted age range of 18–60 years for disc prolapse, it is more often believed to be a condition primarily of young adults – more commonly males and those subject to heavy work.

The controversy that exists between authors arises, at least in part, because of the lack of differentiation made between disc prolapse and disc disease in general. Disc prolapse is the initial pathology after which the disc is diseased for all time, and the effect of altered mechanics or the occurrence of secondary pathology leads to symptoms at a later date in some of the affected patients. In this chapter we are considering the initial disc prolapse when the nucleus protrudes through a rent in the annulus to displace or damage neighbouring tissues. Herniation occurs almost always in one of the two potentially weak points – vertically into the cartilage end-plate or backwards where the posterior segment of the annulus is not only thinner than the anterior and lateral segments, but is also less firmly attached to the bone (Vernon-Roberts, 1976). In central posterior prolapse the disc tissue passes backwards towards the spinal canal by damaging the posterior longitudinal ligament and if large may involve the cauda equina. Much more often the prolapse is posterolateral into the intervertebral foramina to potentially displace or damage ligaments, blood vessels, dura mater or nerve roots. Although some of these tissues are pain-sensitive, for example the posterior longitudinal ligament which can give rise to pain in the back, pressure on nerve roots is of itself not painful but produces paraesthesia.

Macnab (1977) provides evidence that the pain of disc herniation is related to inflammatory reactions around the nerve root, whereas Cyriax (1969) believes that a detached or hinged fragment of annulus produces pain by pressing on the dura mater and in turn this displaced piece of disc can be reduced by manipulation.

Wyke (1976) describes posterolateral herniation impinging initially on the sinuvertebral nerve, in which the protrusion not only interrupts mechano-receptor afferent activity but may also irritate the contained nociceptive afferent fibres and thereby give rise to pain in the lower back in the absence of sciatica. Wyke continues

should the nuclear protrusion develop further, it begins to impinge on the related dorsal nerve roots (and their containing dural sleeves) − as a result of which the backache becomes more severe and more widely distributed (being reinforced by concomitant reflex muscle spasm), and to it are added sensory changes and pain experienced in the distribution of the sciatic nerve.

He also notes that because of the considerable obliquity of the dorsal nerve roots within the lower end of the adult spinal canal, an expanding posterolateral protrusion from the disc between the fourth and fifth lumbar vertebrae impinges not only on the fifth lumbar dorsal root but also involves the first sacral root. Thus irritative compression of the descending branch of the second lumbar nerve within the posterior longitudinal ligament by posterior herniation of the nuclei of one or other of the more rostral lumbar intervertebral discs may give rise to pain experienced in the fifth lumbar dermatomal region of the back. Wyke writes that most frequently herniation occurs between the fourth and fifth lumbar vertebrae and less often between the fifth lumbar and first sacral vertebrae. Although no one would disagree that these are the two levels associated with nearly all disc prolapses, Helfet and Lee (1978) quote 90 per cent of prolapses as occurring between L_5 and S_1 and most of the rest as being at both the L_{4-5} and L_5-S_1 levels.

Macnab (1977) believes that L_5-S_1 prolapses first and is self-limiting whereas L_{4-5} is the 'backache disc'. Cyriax (1969) quotes one in a thousand disc prolapses as being at L_1 or L_2, 4–8 per cent at L_3, 43 per cent at L_4 and 43 per cent at L_5. Although in most cases of disc herniation extruded material comes to lie in a posterolateral position producing unilateral signs and symptoms, Helfet and Lee state that there is often some extension of the prolapse across the midline so that signs are present bilaterally. As the prolapse increases in severity, symptoms change to signs.

The onset of pain is often sudden during bending, twisting or lifting. The pain is agonizing and prevents the patient from standing up. It may be heralded by an audible click. The pattern is usually a minimal provocative incident, or indeed no provocative incident at all, followed by very dramatic symptoms. The patient is locked in flexion, less often in side-flexion, by midline or bilateral lumbar pain. After seconds or minutes he is able to stand but only cautious movements are possible. The pain is aggravated by coughing or sneezing. Radiation occurs to the leg at the same time or shortly thereafter in a sciatic distribution. Sometimes pain in the buttock and down the back of the thigh follows after a few days. As the sciatic pain increases the backache decreases in severity. Pain is aggravated by general and specific activities (such as, bending, stooping, lifting and straining at stool) and relieved by recumbency. Atypical cases are very common. The pain is sometimes of gradual onset and radiation may be absent. Cyriax (1969) divides cases with delayed pain occurring hours after stooping or lifting into a group to which he attributes nuclear herniation instead of the more usual annular herniation. Jayson (1978) refers to two types of referred pain — pressure on ligaments, etc. producing dull pain in muscles at the same embryonic level, and nerve root damage which is well localized with numbness and paraesthesiae. Although pain is more marked proximally, numbness and tingling are more common in the leg and foot.

Patients present with a rigid spine and a loss of the normal lumbar lordosis. There may be a lumbar scoliosis or segmental kyphosis due to spasm of the paraspinal muscles. Helfet and Lee (1978) describe a pathognomonic alternating scoliosis, in which the patient adopts a unilateral sciatic tilt with spasm but can be persuaded by the examiner to straighten the tilt, with increasing difficulty until the back suddenly tilts to the opposite side. This deformity is said to be probably due to incarceration of a nerve root on one side. As the back is extending, the prolapsed portion of the disc squeezes the nerve root even tighter until the root suddenly slips over the fibrous lump and ends on the other side.

Some arcs of movement are normal whereas others are markedly reduced. Forward flexion is greatly restricted, as may be extension also. The patient often leans towards the side of the pain on bending forwards. Lateral flexion is usually relatively pain-free and rotation may be normal in one or even both directions. Straight leg raising is reduced in nearly all cases whereas cross-leg pain is pathognomonic of severe disc prolapse. There may be sensory loss, motor weakness or impairment of tendon jerks. Sensory loss, unlike pain, may be of localizing value and standard texts provide tables of nerve root levels equated against such losses. A central prolapse may damage the cauda equina with pain, paraesthesia and sensory loss in the low back, buttocks, perineum and lower limbs. There may be interference with micturition and defaecation and such cases must be dealt with as surgical emergencies.

Radiographs are normal or show disc space narrowing and are useful only for the exclusion of serious pathology. Jayson (1978) sets out well the indications for myelography, radiculography, epidural myelography, vertebral venography and discography.

The treatment of acute disc prolapse is bedrest and analgesics. If symptoms have not abated or have worsened after 2 weeks, alternative medical or surgical measures must be contemplated. More often some improvement will have taken place and further improvement is to be expected over the ensuing weeks. Unfortunately subsequent episodes of back pain are almost the rule – the mechanism of these will be described below.

IN SUMMARY

79.   Acute prolapsed intervertebral disc occurs in young adults, usually males undergoing heavy work. Herniation occurs vertically into the cartilage end-plate or backwards.

80.   Posterior herniations are either central or posterolateral. Central prolapses may involve the cauda equina with sensory signs in the perineum and interference with micturition and defaecation. They must be treated as surgical emergencies.

81.   Posterolateral herniations produce back pain and radiating sciatic pain by displacing or damaging pressure-sensitive tissues. Almost all prolapses occur between L_4 and L_5 or between L_5 and S_1.

82.   Sudden, agonizing pain is often precipitated by an awkward lift and twist. Patients present with a rigid spine and gross loss of forward flexion. Straight-leg raising is reduced and there may be sensory loss, motor weakness or impairment of tendon jerks.

83.   Radiographs are normal and are only useful to exclude other pathology. Treatment is bedrest and analgesics.

14 Osteoarthritis of the facet joints

The displaced nuclear material from a disc prolapse heals by fibrosis and shrinkage. This reduces the thickness of the disc and is represented in radiographs as joint space narrowing. The relationship between adjacent vertebrae has been described at great length in this monograph to emphasize that the intervertebral disc cannot be regarded in isolation, but as part of a complex arrangement between vertebrae involving also the two posterior intervertebral joints (apophyseal or facet joints) and various ligaments. The whole is a dynamic system allowing movement to take place in a controlled manner between two vertebrae in eight directions – a situation quite different from the concept that regards the disc only as a shock-absorber for compressive forces. As Cyriax (1969) explains, the ankle joint is subject to more of the body mass than individual vertebrae yet manages extremely well without a shock-absorbing disc. As the disc, facet joints and ligaments function together, a derangement of one sooner or later affects the others. Kapandji's diagram (1974) is well worth repeating as it shows one of the mechanisms said to connect the individual functions of the various units making up the total joint between adjacent vertebrae (Figure **14.1**).

The superior vertebra pivots about the fulcrum formed by the facet joints (1) on the inferior vertebra so that tension in the posterior (interspinous) ligament (3) helps the compressive resistance of the disc to withstand compressive forces. Already the effects of disc height narrowing can be seen – in the static situation the posterior ligaments are stretched, either giving rise to pain or resulting in ligamentous dysfunction.

In dynamic situations, movements between the vertebrae will be restricted, especially forward flexion, and the facet joints will be forced to articulate in non-physiological positions of the articular surfaces. In the model that proposes the spine to consist of three vertical pillars, the

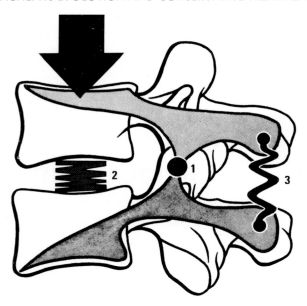

Figure 14.1 Lever system of vertebra (from Kapandji, 1974)

derangement of one of these (the pillar composed of vertebral bodies and discs) will lead to greater demands on the other two (left and right pillars of articular processes and joints). It is not surprising that a combination of these factors leads to wear and tear of the articular surfaces of the facet joints – a process that begins as soon as the disc shrinks and may take 20 years or more to be seen in radiographs. The relative importance of wear and tear compared to hereditary, immunological and biochemical factors in the development of osteoarthritis of the facet joints is often debated. Osteoarthritis certainly can occur in the absence of disc prolapse if another part of the functional unit, for example the ligaments, are damaged or malfunction. There may be an inherent abnormality present in the facet joints themselves predisposing the formation of osteoarthritic changes and examples of these are described below. They may be either congenital malformations or injuries. Even disease involving the cartilage end-plates of the vertebral bodies can lead to degenerative spondylosis (that is, degeneration of the disc and osteoarthritis of the apophyseal joints). Whatever the aetiology of the changes, radiographic evidence can be seen at the age of 50 in 80 per cent of males and 60 per cent of females and at the age of 70 in virtually all radiographs (Schmorl and Junghanns, 1971). The condition is found more commonly, like disc prolapse, in those subject to heavy work. All accounts of the clinical picture emphasize that despite marked radiological evidence of spondylosis, many subjects do not have any major symptoms.

The pathology consists of degeneration of the body-to-body (disc) joints with disc narrowing and a loss of the distinction between nucleus and annulus. There is hypertrophy of bone at the vertebral rims leading to the formation of osteophytes. The changes of osteoarthritis in the facet joints are identical to osteoarthritis in any diarthrodial joint – attrition of the articular cartilage, sclerosis of articular bone and the production of osteophytic spurs at the joint margins which encroach on the intervertebral foramina. The changes in the facet joints are probably the more important from a clinical point of view (Adams, 1971).

Patients complain, if at all, of a local aching pain principally in the low back. The pain is worse during activity and sometimes radiates into the lower limb. In the lumbar area pain tends to occur in acute exacerbations which arise suddenly and last a few weeks. Symptoms may arise from a partial tear of a ligament, subluxation or locking of an unstable degenerate joint or overlying muscle spasm. Spinal movements are moderately restricted, especially forward flexion. Straight leg raising may be limited. Haematological and biochemical investigations are normal.

Radiographs show disc space narrowing with sclerosis of the bone ends and osteophytes around the margins of the vertebral end-plates. There may be gas within the disc. Later there are changes in the facet joints which are best seen in oblique projections – joint space narrowing and sharpening of the margins of the facets, perhaps with osteophytes which may protrude into the intervertebral foramina. Apophyseal osteoarthritis can be seen radiographically in the absence of symptoms, and Lawrence, Bremner, and Brier (1966) found little relation between these X-ray changes and back pain.

IN SUMMARY

84.   A disc prolapse heals by shrinkage and reduces the thickness of the disc. The disc is only one part of the complex arrangement between vertebrae allowing controlled movement in all directions, so derangement of this part sooner or later affects the other parts (the facet joints and posterior ligaments).

85.   The altered mechanics lead to osteoarthritis of the facet joints although the same condition can occur if another part of the functional unit, for example the ligaments, malfunction. The wear and tear starts as soon as the disc has prolapsed in early middle age and progresses over the next 20 or more years.

86.   Radiographic evidence of these changes can be seen in 75 per cent of the population aged 50 years or more but X-ray changes are not always associated with symptoms.

87.   Symptoms occur in acute exacerbations which arise suddenly and last a few weeks. Patients complain of a local aching pain in the low back, sometimes radiating to the lower limb. Haematological and biochemical investigations are normal.

15 Facet joint malfunction

The extent to which the facet joints are involved in the production of low back pain is one of the most widely debated topics in this branch of medicine. Some deny that facet joint pathology is ever a cause of backache whilst others cite these lesions in the majority of cases. The interdependence of apophyseal joints, discs and ligaments has been described and it is usually impossible to identify the exact site contributing to the pain. It is usually safer to ascribe symptoms to mechanical derangements of a general nature rather than specifying a condition such as 'locking' of facet joints or 'blocks', the existence of which can only remain speculative. Jayson (1978) casts the same doubt upon subluxations of the apophyseal joints, pointing out that neither microscopic nor macroscopic evidence of such changes has been demonstrated in these joints. On the other hand Adams (1971) describes momentary subluxation, with consequent ligamentous strain in an intervertebral joint that is unstable on account of disc degeneration or osteo-arthritis, as a cause of acute lumbago (which he denotes as a syndrome of sudden, agonizing pain in the lumbar region, usually occurring on stooping, lifting, turning or coughing). Reilly *et al.*, writing in Helfet and Lee (1978), suggest that 'chiropractic manipulations work by reducing minor subluxations of a lax posterior joint. This laxity would also explain the tendency to recurrent episodes of low back pain.' They advocate that

the most minor strains produce synovitis of one or both posterior joints. When the synovium is torn, haemarthrosis results. On the side where tension is exerted there may be a tear of the capsule and a posterior joint with a lax capsule subject to further strain. Small fragments of articular cartilage and underlying bone may be broken off the joint surface and form loose bodies, which are responsible for recurrent or chronic pain (Harris and Macnab, 1954).

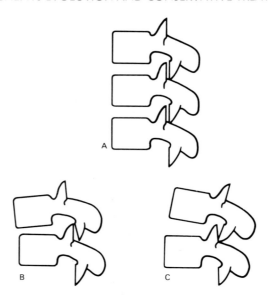

Figure 15.1   In the early stages of degenerative disc disease, excessive degrees of flexion and extension are permitted at the involved segment. This abnormal mobility is associated with rocking of the posterior joints (B and C) (from Macnab, 1977)

Macnab (1977), writing in his own book, gives an excellent account of segmental instability and its sequelae. Segmental instability occurs when the normal movement between vertebrae is lost because of degenerative changes involving any one of the components of the disc. Excessive degrees of flexion and extension are permitted and a certain amount of backward and forward gliding movements occur as well (Figure **15.1**). Macnab (1977) believes instability by itself is probably not painful, but the spine becomes vulnerable to trauma. He writes

A forced and unguarded movement may be concentrated on the wobbly segment and produce a posterior joint strain or a posterior joint subluxation. Repeated injuries may indeed produce osteochondral fractures and loose bodies in the posterior joints.

The next stage of disc degeneration is segmental hyperextension. Extension of the lumbar spine is limited by the anterior fibers of the annulus. When degenerative changes cause these fibers to lose their elasticity, the involved segment or segments may hyperextend.

A similar change may be seen in the next stage of disc degeneration, disc narrowing. As the intervertebral discs lose height, the posterior joints must override and subluxate. In both segmental hyperextension and disc narrowing, the related posterior joints in normal posture are held in hyperextension, and this postural defect is exaggerated if the patient has weak abdominal muscles and/or tight tensors, is overweight, is overwrought, and wears high heels – the typical North American housewife after four pregnancies.

When the posterior joints are held at the extreme of their limit of extension, there is no safety factor of movement and the extension strains of everyday living may push the joints past their physiologically permitted limits and thereby produce pain. Eventually the posterior joints may subluxate.

This sequence is shown in Figure **15.2**.

Thus the consensus of expert opinion is in favour of the existence of posterior joint subluxation, and if this opinion is correct it may explain the empirical evidence obtained from clinical trials of spinal manipulation (see later) which indicate that manipulation is effective in patients aged 45 years or more. One can easily imagine disc degeneration in early middle-age giving rise to mechanical instability which renders the spine vulnerable to trauma, as a result of which pain may arise from ligamentous or posterior joint damage. The latter leads to posterior joint subluxation which is corrected by manipulation. If the vertebral body–disc–body union is involved earlier in life (for example in adolescents with Scheuermann's

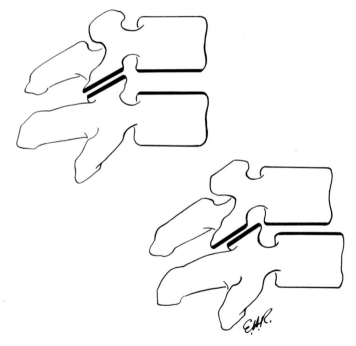

Figure 15.2 As the intervertebral discs lose height and the vertebral bodies approach one another, the posterior joints must override and assume the position normally held in hyperextension. It is to be noted that owing to the inclination of the posterior joints, as the upper vertebral body approaches the vertebral body beneath it, it is displaced backwards producing a retrospondylolisthesis. This posterior displacement of the vertebral body, indicative of posterior joint subluxation, is readily recognizable on routine X-ray examination of the lumbar spine. (from Macnab, 1977)

syndrome), facet joint pathology occurs that much earlier (early 30s) and although subluxation can be corrected by manipulation, the ligaments are so lax that relief is only temporary and the subluxation recurs within a matter of weeks or even days.

Subluxation is not the only possibility when considering the apophyseal joints as a source of back pain. Fractures of the apophyseal joints may be more common than formerly imagined. In seven patients Sims-Williams, Jayson, and Baddeley (1978) identified only one fracture on conventional anteroposterior and lateral films, and a second fracture on oblique views; but stereovision revealed fractures in all seven. In this technique the stereo-plotter allows the apophyseal joints to be examined with greater precision using binocular stereovision. The authors believed that these small fractures were due to repeated minor stresses in the bone with eventual fatigue failure in the laminae and apophyseal facets. Wiltse, Widdell, and Jackson (1975) thought that such fatigue fractures are responsible for most cases of spondylosis and spondylolytic spondylolisthesis. Shah et al. (1976) have shown that there is a greater concentration of strain in the posterior elements of the spine than in the anterior elements and that these strains are increased by extension. The areas of strain concentration corresponded closely with the sites of fractures found in the patients of Sims-Williams et al. The fractures also resembled those described by Farfan (1973) when axial compression loading was used to fracture the lamina and inferior articular processes of degenerate joints.

It is also possible that, as Harris and Macnab (1954) describe, the articular surface of the apophyseal joints become frayed and pieces flake off. Occasionally quite large osteochondral fractures are found. As in other joints these fragments may form loose bodies which lie free in the joint or become secondarily attached to the synovial membrane (Lancet, 1978). Apophyseal arthritis was described in the previous chapter. The arthritic facet joints, like joints of the extremities, exhibit a mixture of degenerative and restorative processes. Osteophytes in the lumbar spine have long been implicated as irritants to the spinal nerve roots as they course out through the intervertebral foramina. In an adult the intervertebral foramen has approximately five to six times the diameter of the nerve which courses through it (Maslow and Rothman, 1975). However in both flexion and extension of the lumbar spine the available space decreases markedly, and it is the facets which cause this compromise of available space. Pressure on the nerves may be further aggravated by osteophytes projecting into the intervertebral foramina from the margins of osteoarthritic apophyseal joints (Vernon-Roberts, 1976).

Apart from pressure on spinal nerve roots, the nociceptive receptor system in the capsules of the apophyseal joints may be excited by abnormal forces during movement (Wyke, 1976). It is not difficult to imagine sublux-ation producing the same capsular stretching with resultant pain. The capsule of the intervertebral joint has three kinds of pain receptor; it includes complex unencapsulated and small encapsulated endings as well as the more usual free-fibre endings (Maslow and Rothman, 1975). There is empirical evidence that arthritic changes in the facet joint causes pain in the back. Injection of local anaesthetics into the joint eases some back pain and surgical fusion eliminates movement and sometimes eliminates pain. A number of studies have shown that painful stimuli in the dorsal structures of the spine — in the area innervated by the dorsal ramus — can cause referred pain in the leg in a region innervated by the anterior ramus. Mooney and Robertson (1976) found that injection of irritant fluid precisely in the apophyseal joint caused referred pain patterns indistinguishable from that associated with a prolapsed disc. Furthermore, because irritation of the receptor system in the lumbar apophyseal joint capsules may give rise to reflex spasm of the paravertebral musculature, such patients may also complain of pain (and indicate tenderness) in the deep soft tissues lateral to the lumbar spine (Wyke, 1976).

With apophyseal joint pathology producing on occasions back pain, referred pain and reflex spasm of muscles, it is perhaps prudent that this chapter started with a warning not to diagnose lesions of these joints on purely clinical grounds.

IN SUMMARY

88. The facet joints are subject to small fractures which may remain undetected unless a binocular stereoplotter is used. These fractures are believed to be due to repeated minor stresses in the bone with eventual fatigue failure in the laminae and apophyseal facets.

89. Many authors describe subluxations of facet joints and some believe that manipulation works by reducing these minor subluxations. Clinical trials have shown manipulation to be efficacious in patients aged 45 years or more — an age when apophyseal joint pathology would be expected to occur secondary to pre-existing disc degeneration.

90. Facet joint pathology produces neurological symptoms in two ways. Firstly, osteophytes or subluxed facets encroach upon the intervertebral foramen causing pressure on spinal nerve roots. Secondly, the joint capsule itself is stretched by excessive movements and the contained nerve endings give rise to pain.

91. Studies have shown that these dorsal structures lead to back pain, referred pain in the leg and spasm of the overlying muscles. Apart from the age at which facet joint pathology produces symptoms, and the techniques which possibly ablate these symptoms, the clinical picture (as outlined in item 87) is indistinguishable from that caused by lesions of neighbouring tissues.

16 Lesions of ligaments

Whereas muscles act to produce movement about joints, ligaments stabilize joints and control the degree of movement that takes place. They are capable only of withstanding tensile forces but the anterior longitudinal ligament, for example, has double the tensile strength of the cancellous bone of the vertebral body (Shah, 1976). If a ligament ruptures, movement about the joint is excessive in the directions normally limited by that ligament. Complete rupture of a ligament produces a brief sensation of snapping accompanied by a stab of pain at the time of the injury, but the predominant symptom is loss of function and the ensuing pain may be minimal. For example, surgical disruption of the supraspinous ligament does not lead to the development of low back pain, so Macnab (1977) believes segmental instability is responsible for the symptoms. A sprained ligament is a partial tear which is felt as an immediate pain after lifting or twisting. Usually it is followed by a pain-free interval after which the patient develops stiffness that limits his mobility. The stiffness subsides over a few days.

Like the capsules of the related apophyseal and sacroiliac joints, the ligaments and their attached aponeuroses are richly innervated by nociceptive nerve endings. Wyke (1976) believes that backache is readily produced from these tissues when they are subjected to abnormal mechanical stresses (as by prolonged standing, especially while wearing high-heeled shoes; by persistently distorted postures in occupational circumstances, or as a result of structural abnormalities of the vertebral column; or by attempts to lift or support heavy weights). Macnab emphasizes that the supraspinous ligament can give rise not only to back pain but also to referred pain as shown by the injection of hypertonic saline into the lumbosacral supraspinous ligament which may give rise to pain radiating down the leg as far as

167

the calf, and may also be associated with tender points commonly situated over the sacroiliac joint and the upper outer quadrant of the buttock. On the other hand, Wyke believes that because of the diffuse distribution of the receptor system through the vertebral connective tissues and because of the widespread intersegmental linkages between their afferent nerve fibres, attempts to use such a procedure as a means of delineating a supposed segmental nociceptive innervation of the spinal tissues are clearly fallacious.

Already in this chapter the two mechanisms by which the ligaments can be cited in the production of low back pain have become evident. Firstly, damaged ligaments add to *segmental instability*, and secondly, ligaments may be affected by persistently distorted postures when they are subject to *abnormal mechanical stresses.*

Segmental instability is a logical progression from the disc degeneration and facet joint pathology described in the previous chapters. Kapandji's diagram (1974) (Figure **14.1**) shows that the posterior ligaments are stretched when the intervertebral disc thickness is reduced in the same way that removing clothes from a clothes-peg increases the distance between the handles. Tearing of the supraspinous ligament can only occur in the presence of disc degeneration allowing an abnormal degree of flexion or with an injury severe enough to disrupt the posterior fibres of the annulus and the capsule of the posterior joints (Macnab, 1977). Lumbar instability is secondary to disease and injury of the discs, osteoarthritis and traumatic rupture of ligaments with or without fracture. It occurs in the young only after severe trauma, but in the middle-aged and older patients as a long-term result of trauma or in degenerative conditions. With advancing age the elasticity of the ligaments is decreased (as it is as a result of hormonal changes associated with ingestion of oestogen-containing oral contraceptive agents or with developing pregnancy). In spite of the differences described by Helfet and Lee (1978) between the clinical features of disc prolapse and segmental instability, the two are extremely similar and, of course, often occur together. Pure ligamentous disease tends not to lead to pain on coughing and sneezing, straight leg raising is not limited and neurological signs are usually absent. In addition it is usually written that with ligamentous lesions spinal movements are full, even if painful, as long as a disc lesion or facet joint lesion is not present.

Abnormal mechanical stresses are responsible for the chronic lower lumbar ligamentous strain or postural back pain as described by Adams (1971). Unlike lumbar instability which occurs mainly in the middle-aged and older patients, postural back pain occurs in the young and middle-aged. The patient is nearly always a woman. There is a history of long-continued lumbar or lumbosacral backache with a total lack of clinical or radiological abnormalities. Aching persists for many years and is a source of nagging discomfort rather than a serious handicap. It is worse on prolonged standing, especially combined with leaning forwards, and aggravated by wearing high-heeled shoes. Whereas segmental instability leads to strains in the posterior lumbar ligaments, postural back pain arises from the sacroiliac ligaments and the iliolumbar ligaments. With a loss of tone in the abdominal muscles (for example, during pregnancy) the pelvis tends to rotate forwards due to the weight of the abdominal contents. The sacroiliac ligaments stop the pelvis from rotating forwards on the sacrum; once the sacroiliac joint is fixed, the iliolumbar ligaments resist the forward rotation of the pelvis plus sacrum, and with this rotation, lordosis is increased. The whole picture is one of weak abdominal muscles, forward pelvic rotation, tension in sacro-iliac and iliolumbar ligaments and increased lumbar lordosis.

For many years French clinicians have recognized that long periods in poorly designed working conditions may lead to postural backache in young women with hypermobile spines (Chabot, 1962). Swedish workers (Hirsch, Jonsson, and Lewin, 1969) have described a condition of 'low back insufficiency' which comprises over half the women with back symptoms and the majority of the younger patients (15–24 years). These patients had a history of repeated attacks of lumbar pain without sciatica. The presence of hypermobility was not reported but the group was mutually exclusive of another group who complained of intensive localized pain and had limited movements. Howes and Isdale (1971) described the 'loose back syndrome' and showed that women exhibiting both spinal and peripheral ligamentous laxity comprised more than half a group of consecutive female cases of 'problem' backache seen in consultation. The syndrome was only seen in a small number of male cases of 'problem' backache and in correlating the clinical diagnosis and the analysis of joint movement findings, there was a striking difference between the men and the women. The authors suggested that this is an important differential diagnosis of backache in women.

IN SUMMARY

92. Segmental instability is a logical progression from the disc degener-ation and facet joint pathology described in the previous chapters and needs only failure of the posterior vertebral ligaments. It occurs in the young only after severe trauma but in the middle-aged and older patients as a long-term result of trauma or in degenerative conditions.

93. As the ligamentous pathology usually occurs as part of a whole-joint syndrome, symptoms are indistinguishable from facet joint lesions. If the ligaments are involved alone, spinal movements are full and signs of both dural irritation and neurological involvement are absent.

94. The second mechanism by which ligaments are involved in low back pain concerns chronic lower lumbar ligamentous strain or postural backache. This is a prolonged, low-degree ache in young women,

associated with hypermobility and a total lack of clinical or radio-logical abnormalities.

95.   The picture is one of weak abdominal muscles, forward pelvic rotation, tension in the sacroiliac and iliolumbar ligaments and increased lumbar lordosis. This syndrome may be responsible for half of the cases of low back pain in young women.

17 Spondylolysis and spondylolisthesis

The segmental instability which follows as a result of disc degeneration and partial ligamentous failure sometimes produces a special type of lesion in the lower lumbar spine, commonly at the L_4 level. Excessive mobility on flexion and extension contributes towards degenerative changes in the posterior joints which in turn allows forward and backward gliding of the involved vertebral bodies. Subluxation of the arthritic apophyseal joints permits forward displacement of one vertebral body on the adjacent vertebra below, and the displacement becomes fixed because of an increase in the angle between the pedicle and the inferior processes (Macnab, 1977) (Figure **17.1**).

The forward slip of L_4 on L_5 is never very great but occasionally root entrapment may be produced by a combination of annular bulge, buckling of the ligamentum flavum and subluxation of the posterior joints which are enlarged by osteophytic outgrowths. Thus disc degeneration, gross segmental instability and posterior joint damage predispose to this condition which is found predominantly in females with an average age of about 50 years. It is known as degenerative spondylolisthesis and occurs without any accompanying defect in the neural arch. The historical literature on spondylolisthesis focused interest on the neural arch defect to such an extent that the possibility of forward displacement with an intact neural arch was obscured. Macnab believes that one form of isthmic spondylolisthesis has a break in the pars interarticularis which is secondary to the vertebral slip and is not the cause of it. The basic lesion is said to be the stretching-out of the pars interarticularis as though it were made of plastic (Figure **17.2**).

Because there is no defect in the pars interarticularis, the neural arch comes forward with the slipping vertebra. The degree of slip is usually quite marked and the cauda equina may be compressed between the laminae of

171

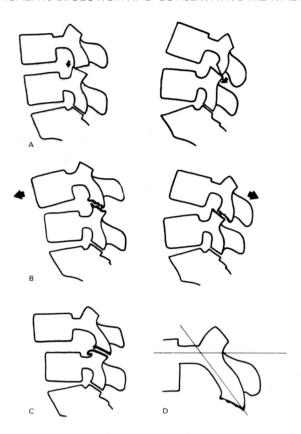

Figure 17.1   Mechanical insufficiency of an intervertebral disc permits excessive movement on flexion and extension (A). The posterior joints undergo degenerative changes because of this abnormal movement and with increasing breakdown permit forward and backward gliding of the involved vertebral bodies (B). Subluxation of the arthritic zygapophysial joints permits forward displacement of the vertebral body (C), and the displacement becomes fixed because of an increase in the angle between the pedicle and the inferior processes (D) (from Macnab, 1977)

L_4 and L_5 and the dorsal area of the first sacral body. However the majority of patients have no evidence of nerve root compression because the isthmus is sufficiently elongated. The average age for onset of symptoms is about 15 years and the patient presents complaining of a sudden onset of backache and has a rigid lumbar spine commonly associated with scoliosis. The pelvis is rotated anteriorly, giving rise to a flat sacrum; hamstring spasm is frequently seen, making the patient walk with bent knees (Macnab, 1977).

Wiltse, Widdell, and Jackson (1975) contend that, except for the occasional acute fractures of the pars interarticularis, all cases of isthmic

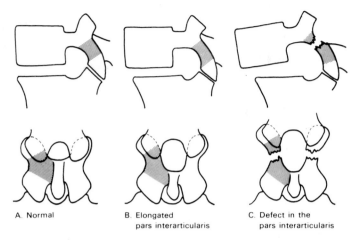

A. Normal

B. Elongated
pars interarticularis

C. Defect in the
pars interarticularis

Figure 17.2   Isthmic spondylolisthesis. The pars interarticularis which was normal at birth (A) becomes attenuated and elongated allowing the vertebral body to slip forwards in relationship to the vertebral body below (B). Eventually on some occasions, the elongated pars interarticularis may break (C). This defect in the pars interarticularis is, however, secondary to the slip and is not the cause of the forward displacement of the vertebral body (from Macnab, 1977)

spondylolysis or spondylolisthesis begin as fatigue fractures, and they interpret their cases of elongated but intact pars interarticularis as instances of an unusual manifestation of the healing process of fatigue fractures. The healing may result from repeated cracking and healing of the pars interarticularis, each time with slightly more elongation.

Whereas spondylolisthesis is defined as forward slipping of a vertebral body on the one below it, spondylolysis is defined as a defect in the pars interarticularis without vertebral slipping. There is loss of bony continuity between the superior and inferior articular processes, the deficiency being bridged by fibrous tissue. Neural arch defects occur most commonly between the ages of 5 and 7 years. The sudden increase in incidence at this age has always been difficult to explain, for the condition is unusual in 5-year-old children yet the prevalence is 5 per cent in 7-year-olds. Thus a condition that was originally thought to be congenital became regarded as one caused by injury or stress fracture. Wiltse, Widdell, and Jackson (1975) studied those cases developing between the age of 7 and adulthood and showed that the basic lesion was the result of repeated trauma and fatigue fracture rather than acute fractures.

The fatigue fractures may have a strong hereditary basis and the incidence seems to be higher than generally appreciated in children and adolescents with low back pain and paraspinal muscle spasm. Defects are much more commonly found in boys than in girls, and this fact may be related to the more violent physical activity of boys as compared with girls. Wiltse *et al.* list the respects in which the fine linear defect in the pars interarticularis differs from other fatigue fractures as:

(1) It tends to develop at an earlier age than other fatigue fractures.

(2) There is a hereditary disposition.

(3) The fluffy periosteal callus formation so often seen in other fatigue fractures is seen only occasionally. When this type of callus is seen, it is usually in the 18 or 19-year-old who has subjected his back to the stresses of a long march while carrying a pack.

(4) In contrast to the usual fatigue fracture in a long bone that develops during unaccustomed repetitive stress, at least in the 5–7-year-old child, this lesion seems to develop following rather minor trauma. Virtually no patient at this age is aware that the lesion is developing.

(5) The defect in the pars interarticularis tends to persist, whereas fatigue fractures in other bones virtually always heal.

Healing of the defect can occur even in the absence of treatment without anyone knowing that the lesion was ever present. Much more frequently it remains a pseudarthrosis and in some studies vertebral slippage or spondylolisthesis developed about 50 per cent of the time. Forward slipping of the vertebral body occurs most frequently between the ages of 10 and 15 years and rarely increases after 20.

A defect in the pars interarticularis is the most common lesion in spondylolisthesis in people below the age of 50. Approximately 6 per cent of the white population of the United States was reported to have this defect. Its incidence varies considerably with race, being about one-third as frequent in blacks as in whites, and reaching as high as 60 per cent in some isolated Eskimo communities in the far north. It is most unlikely that this percentage of affected individuals is severely handicapped by low back pain, and the incidence of the condition has not been found to be significantly greater in adult patients with low back pain compared to the population as a whole. Thus one must question how often neural arch defects are a source of symptoms. Macnab (1977) believes that if the X-ray of a patient with back pain shows a spondylolisthesis, the defect is probably the cause of the symptoms if the patient is under 26, possibly the cause if the patient is between 26 and 40 and rarely the cause if the patient is over 40. In spondylolytic spondylolisthesis a forward slip of more than 50 per cent is frequently associated with hyperlordosis and this may be responsible for part or all of the symptoms. Symptoms attributable to the spondylolytic spondylolisthesis are of back pain and stiffness related to posture. The altered positions of the vertebrae may trap nerve roots, producing root symptoms. Once more we see a condition thought to be due to repetitive trauma (spondylolytic spondylolisthesis) occurring more commonly in males, and a condition due to excessive mobility and instability (degenerative spondylolisthesis) occurring more commonly in females.

IN SUMMARY

96. Vertebral segmental instability permits excessive flexion and extension which in turn contributes towards further degenerative changes in the posterior facet joints. Forward and backward gliding of the involved vertebrae ensues until one vertebra (often L_4 in degenerative spondylolisthesis) becomes fixed in a forward displacement on the vertebra below. This condition, like many others in which hypermobility is a predisposing feature, is more common in females and the average age of onset is about 50 years.

97. In younger patients this forward slippage of one vertebra on the one below (spondylolisthesis) nearly always follows a defect in the pars interarticularis (spondylolysis). The neural arch defects occur most commonly between the ages of 5 and 7 years, the sudden increase in incidence at this age remaining unexplained. The cases developing between the ages of 7 years and adulthood have been shown to be due to repeated trauma causing fatigue fractures. More energetic physical activity may explain the higher incidence in boys than in girls. The fatigue fractures develop in persons with a hereditary disposition and tend to persist.

98. In about 50 per cent of cases of spondylolysis, forward slipping of the vertebral body eventually occurs, most frequently between the ages of 10 and 15 years. Of the white population of the United States 6 per cent have the defect in the pars interarticularis and often the condition is symptomless. If the X-ray of a patient with back pain shows a spondylolisthesis, the defect is probably the cause of the symptoms if the patient is under 26, possibly the cause if the patient is between 26 and 40 and rarely the cause if the patient is over 40 (Macnab, 1977).

18 The sacroiliac joint

Many old editions of *Gray's Anatomy* described the sacroiliac joint as diarthrodial but partly united by patches of soft fibrocartilage and fine interosseous fibres. Later editions described it as being a synovial joint marked by a number of irregular elevations and depressions, providing a locking device restricting movement and contributing to the stability of the joint. Only in the elderly, and particularly in the male, is it usual to find that the joint cavity is at least partly obliterated by the presence of fibrous or fibrocartilaginous adhesions. This change of attitude ascribing a certain amount of movement to the joint followed reports in the 1920s which clearly showed movement of a gliding and rotatory nature. By the 1950s Weisl (1955) had investigated the movements of the sacroiliac joint by radiographic methods in the living subject. He identified the axis of rotation and showed that its site was variable. Pitkin and Pheasant (1936) described the movement of the ilia about the symphysis pubis causing torsion of the pelvis thought to occur during walking. The innominate on one side is rotated backwards on the sacrum and that on the other side, forwards. In order for this movement to take place, some twisting must take place at the symphysis pubis. As the range of movement of the sacroiliac joint is small and varies according to the circumstances and to the subject, it is not surprising that there has been little agreement regarding the function of this joint and the significance of its movement. There is no evolutionary evidence from other species of a tendency towards fusion of these joints. Helfet and Lee (1978) believe that the main function of the joint is probably as a shock-absorber, to prevent reactive forces from the limbs reaching the spinal column.

The classical theory of nutation describes rotation between the sacrum and ilium during labour increasing the anteroposterior diameter of the pelvic outlet. This rotation is limited by the sacrotuberous, sacrospinous and anterior sacroiliac ligaments. Various theories advance different sites for the centre of rotation and others describe pure linear displacement rather than rotation. The number of theories available suggests how difficult it is to analyse movements of small range, and raises the possibility that different types of movement may occur in different individuals. Nevertheless the only proven variety of sacroiliac strain is that which follows pregnancy when the sacroiliac joint has opened during delivery and has repositioned incorrectly post partum (Dixon, 1976). Apart from those occurring during the latter months of pregnancy and during labour, sacroiliac strains are rare and need considerable forces such as those generated by falls from heights or motor vehicle injuries. Sacroiliac strain was formerly a common diagnosis in causes of pain localized predominantly in the upper gluteal region. Now it is believed that in the vast majority of such cases the pain does not originate in the sacroiliac joint, but is referred from the lower lumbar spine – often a disc lesion.

During pregnancy the supporting ligaments of the sacroiliac joints become relaxed and the joints are susceptible to strain as a result of even mild trauma. The patients complain of pain localized to the involved sacro-iliac joint; the pain radiates around the greater trochanter and down the anterolateral aspect of the thigh, and is aggravated by twisting the trunk. The diagnosis is not justifiable unless the patient presents, in addition, tender-ness over the symphysis pubis as the pelvis is a closed ring and cannot undergo stretching at one site only. Symptoms experienced clinically may be reproduced on stressing the sacroiliac joint by lateral manual pressure on the iliac crest or by resisted abduction of the hip joint on the affected side. There is a good range of spinal movement on examination with pain only at the extremes. There are no neurological signs. The only radiographic changes are occasional findings of osteitis condensans ilii or the misalign-ment of the two pubic rami at the symphysis. There is no evidence of inflammation or infection in 'osteitis'; the radiographs suggest that the affected area of iliac bone is that which is subject to abnormal weight-bearing due to sacroiliac instability.

Davis and Lentle (1978) showed that it may be possible to find evidence of sacroiliac disease in 25 per cent of women presenting with low back pain if sophisticated scanning techniques are used. Of 22 patients with abnormal scans, 20 had normal radiographs and would have been missed with conventional examinations. Although the underlying factors that lead to this sacroiliac disease are unknown, it seems to be a different entity from classical sacroiliitis of seronegative spondarthritis and does not depend on the same genetic factor. De Roo, Walravens, and Dequeker (1978) question the usefulness of this quantitative sacroiliac scintigraphy in differentiating between control and disease groups on the basis of their experiments with the technique.

IN SUMMARY

99. The sacroiliac joint was formerly considered to be a fused joint without movement. Now movement is believed to exist between the ilia and sacrum.

100. There is little agreement on the type of movement, whether this is by gliding or by rotation and, if the latter, where the centre of rotation is located. The site of this centre might be in different places in different patients and even in the same patient at different times, for example during pregnancy.

101. During pregnancy the relationship between the ilia and sacrum alters to increase the diameter of the pelvic outlet. This phenomenon occurs because the ligaments are relaxed, probably by a hormonal mechanism. The joint on one side may reposition itself incorrectly during the postnatal period. Other than those following labour, sacroiliac strains are rare and follow major trauma.

102. Sacroiliac strain produces pain over the sacroiliac joint which radiates around the greater trochanter and down the anterolateral aspect of the thigh. Manual pressure applied laterally on the iliac crest or resisted abduction of the hip joint reproduce the pain.

103. Sacroiliac disease may be more common than imagined in women and may be present in 25 per cent of those presenting with low back pain.

19 Muscle spasm

Spasm may develop in the muscles of the lower back if there is abnormal activity of the receptors located in the joints of the vertebral column. This can result from posture abnormalities (such as those associated with certain occupations, with the later stages of pregnancy and with prolonged wearing of high-heeled shoes), from mechanical changes in the vertebral column (as with degenerative disc disease or osteoarthritis) or from inflammatory abnormalities in the skeletal and articular tissues of the lumbosacral spine (Wyke, 1976). This reflex hyperactivity of the muscles causes pain by irritating the nerve fibres of intramuscular blood vessels with chemical changes in the interstitial fluid as a result of abnormal metabolic activity. Therefore, muscle spasm is secondary to mechanical derangement of the spine but is responsible for some of the pain experienced by the patient. A vicious circle may exist, with subluxation of the facet joints in the lumbar spine leading to reflex muscle spasm which maintains the joint in its subluxed position. This vicious circle may be broken by abolition of the muscle spasm (for example, by local anaesthetic injection) or by correction of the subluxation (for example, by manipulation).

Unilateral muscle spasm is suggestive of a unilateral posterior joint strain (Helfet and Lee, 1978). Lesions involving both the disc and posterior joints are often accompanied by spasm of the spinal flexors, producing a flat or slightly kyphotic lumbar spine. Psoas spasm produces a flexion deformity of the hip.

Pain in muscles which are tender when gripped or squeezed, especially if firm nodules are felt, is often labelled as fibrositis. This is a clinical rather than a pathological entity for the so-called fibrositic nodules cannot be identified histologically. The aching pain in the posterior spinal muscles is often influenced by climatic changes. The name fibrositis was first introduced by

Sir William Gowers in 1904 to denote non-specific inflammatory changes in fibrous tissue. Macnab (1977) believes that the fibrositic nodules palpable over the iliac crest are usually localized nodules of fat. Because they are situated in an area which is a common site of referred tenderness derived from a spinal lesion, they may be tender on pressure. He quotes the concept of fibrositis ruling supreme as the most common cause of back pain for nearly half a century as a classic example of how the phenomenon of referred pain and tenderness has clouded the recognition of the pathological basis of low back pain derived from soft tissue disorders. There is no reason why the term should not be retained to describe the clinical syndrome of low back pain of undetermined origin associated with tender nodules. However, it should be remembered that the term does not denote a specific pathological process.

This phenomenon of referred pain arises because a deep structure irritated by trauma or disease results in pain which may be experienced locally, referred distally or both. Tenderness may also be referred to a distance. Unlike pain arising from the skin, deep pain is usually diffuse, poorly localized and felt at some distance from the point stimulated. Kellgren (1978) injected intramuscular NaCl to reproduce this steady pain, which lasted for several minutes after the needle was withdrawn, to mark

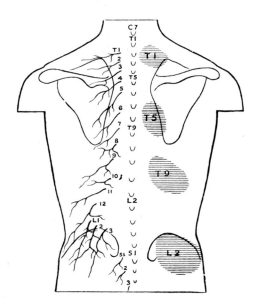

Figure 19.1   On the left the posterior primary divisions of the spinal nerves are shown in their course after piercing the deep fascia. On the right the hatched areas represent some of the corresponding deep pain areas for comparison. (from Kellgren, 1978)

out the distributions of pain from accurately placed stimuli. The skeletal muscles give diffuse pain with distant reference but with a clear segmental distribution. These segmental areas for deep pain differ from the dermatomes which form complete bands round the body. Deep pain often goes through from the back to the front and vice versa. There are one or more areas of maximal pain within the full area and if the pain is slight, only the points of maximal pain will be appreciated. In the trunk these points of maximal pain correspond with the regions where the spinal nerves pierce the deep fascia and give it a rich nerve supply (Figure **19.1**).

Referred tenderness follows the spontaneous pain closely in distribution, time and intensity. The tenderness, like the pain, is not evenly distributed, there being one or more areas of maximal tenderness which are found over the structures normally most sensitive to pressure. The tenderness is rarely severe but always corresponds with the points of maximal spontaneous pain. This phenomenon is quite distinct from the deep tender spot or 'trigger point' which is found in the structure giving rise to the pain. The trigger point frequently lies outside the distribution of the pain, and the patient is not aware of its existence until it is discovered by the physician. Firm pressure on the trigger point produces an increase in referred pain and tenderness together with other reflex phenomena, in fact the whole pain symptom complex; while pressure over areas of maximal referred pain causes increase of pain only. Local anaesthesia of the tigger point from which the pain is arising produces a dramatic and complete abolition of symptoms. Anaesthetizing areas of maximal referred pain abolishes the tenderness and reduces spontaneous pain slightly but any limitation of movement or other disability caused by the pain remains unchanged.

Travell and Rinzler (1952) examined about 1000 patients to identify trigger areas which were defined as small hypersensitive regions from which impulses bombard the central nervous system and give rise to *referred* pain. Pain is produced whenever the trigger area is stimulated by pressure, needling, extreme heat or cold, or motion that stretches the structure containing the trigger area. Trigger mechanisms may be initiated by a variety of stimuli including direct trauma to muscle or joint, chronic muscular strain, chilling of fatigued muscle, arthritis and nerve root injury. A trigger area at a particular spot gives rise to a similar distribution of referred pain in one person as in another. If the trigger point lies in muscle, the muscle can be located by comparing the pain reference pattern with charts in Travell and Rinzler's paper (Figure **19.2**).

Muscles can be involved in low back pain in other ways. Partial tears of muscle attachments may occur in young men as a result of a specific injury. A similar injury sustained by an older man, with weaker muscles and with degenerate discs, is much more likely to result in a posterior joint strain (Macnab, 1977). The local tenderness and pain persist for about 3 weeks, during which time the patient is well advised to avoid provocative activity.

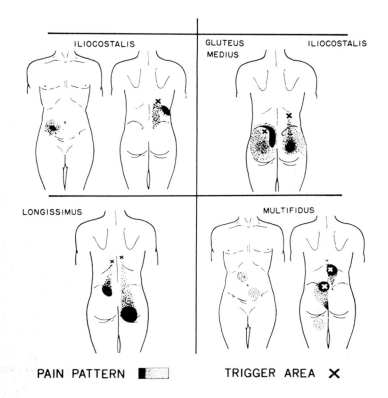

PAIN PATTERN ▉▒░ TRIGGER AREA ✕

Figure 19.2 Trigger areas and referred pain (from Travell and Rinzler, 1952)

Shortening (or tightness) of the hamstrings and biceps surae results from faulty posture due to chronic low back and leg pain. This not uncommon cause of thigh and leg aching must be treated by stretching exercises to restore these muscles to their normal length.

IN SUMMARY

104. An abnormality of a joint in the vertebral column leads to reflex spasm of the muscles in the lower back. Muscle spasm may create a vicious circle by maintaining the abnormality of the joint if this happens to be, for example, a subluxed facet. Muscle spasm is painful because chemical irritants are produced by abnormal metabolic activity.

105. Painful, tender muscles, especially when accompanied by the presence of firm nodules, is sometimes called fibrositis. Formerly this term was thought to denote a specific pathological process but the

nodules cannot be identified histologically. The confusion arose because the muscle pain was referred from an often distant deep structure which was being irritated by trauma or disease.

106.   Referred tenderness accompanies referred pain and both have areas of maximal intensity within the confines of the segment affected.

107.   These points of maximal referred pain are quite distinct from the deep tender spots or trigger points which are found in the structure giving rise to the pain. Stimulation of the trigger point, which often lies outside the painful area, reproduces not only the pain and tenderness but also the other reflex phenomena of the pain symptom complex; pressure over areas of maximal referred pain causes increase in pain only.

20 Muscle fatigue

Wyke (1976) reminds us that everyday experience clearly demonstrates that muscles subjected to prolonged work become fatigued and as a result become locally painful and tender. This applies to the back muscles when they are kept hyperactive by the assumption of persistently distorted standing or sitting postures, or by the demands of occupation or athletic activity. Although the mechanisms involved in the production of muscular fatigue are still not clearly understood they result from biochemical changes that are similar to those in reflex muscle spasm. Despite this, however, the electromyographic appearances presented by fatigued muscles are different from those of muscles involved in reflex spasm, and this is a matter of practical importance in the clinical differential diagnosis of muscular low back pain and its treatment. Muscular fatigue may be relieved by resting the affected muscles and by adopting measures that promote muscle blood flow such as massage and the local application of heat. However, Wyke notes that not all the backache associated with postural or occupational fatigue is derived from the back muscles for part of it comes from the lumbar spinal ligaments and apophyseal joints.

When the forward stooped position is maintained the sacrospinales act as a bowstring to support the spine. In this position the lumbar spine is hyper-extended. Pain not only arises from muscle fatigue of the sacrospinales but, if there is disc space narrowing, from nerve root compression which may be increased (Figure **20.1**).

A third source of pain is provided by spinal ligaments which are continu-ally stretched posterior to the vertebral bodies in the thoracolumbar junction and anterior to the vertebral bodies in the lumbar region. It should be remembered that experimental injection of hypertonic saline into the supraspinous ligaments at $T_{12}-L_1$ gives rise to pain referred to the low back,

187

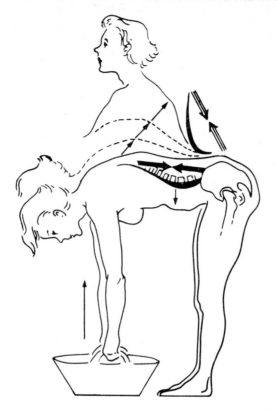

Figure 20.1   When a patient bends forward with the knees straight and then tries to lift, the sacrospinales, when contracting, act as a bowstring and hyperextend the lumbar spine. (from Macnab, 1977)

radiating on occasion to the buttock (Macnab, 1977). Bending forwards, as when stooping over the washbasin or when making beds, can also strain the sacrospinous, sacrotuberous and anterior sacroiliac ligaments which prevent the sacrum from rotating forwards between the two sides of the pelvis.

Ligaments can also be stretched by hyperextension of the spine in the sitting position. Sitting in a theatre with the knees out straight and the floor sloping away will apply a significant extension strain to the spine and the patients tend to irritate the patrons in the row in front by putting their feet on the back of their seat in order to keep their knees and hips flexed. Similarly sitting in a car with the knees held straight hyperextends the spine and prolonged driving is uncomfortable.

Sitting 'up straight' also causes back discomfort by maintaining the hyperlordosis. Females have more social restrictions upon their sitting posture than do males. After all, writes Williams (1974), slumping, leg-crossing and other comfortable positions are 'definitely not ladylike'.

Although standing would seem to be a relatively simple and painless activity, fatigue occurs in the muscles of the low back, for these are the muscles that have been supporting most of the body weight. The electromyographic studies confirming this have been described above. In the process of relaxing the back muscles, the weight is usually shifted backwards onto the heels. High heels increase the problem because they cause the body to tilt forward and even fall unless the trunk is bent backwards to counteract the downward pull of gravity. Obese individuals, as well as pregnant women, both carry an extra load in front for which some backward compensation must be made.

These positions can be avoided by the Williams' axiom: 'Always sit, stand, walk and lie in a way that reduces the hollow in the low back to a minimum'. When these patients stand for long periods of time, the lumbar spine sags into extension and the patients automatically try to flatten the lumbar spine by flexing one hip and knee, as in the act of putting one foot on the seat of a chair or on a bar rail.

Whereas the sacrospinales increase the degree of lordosis, the abdominal muscles and the gluteal muscles flatten the lumbar spine by pulling up on the front of the pelvis and down on the back of the pelvis respectively (Figure **6.20**, page 82). Although the abdominal muscles oppose the erectores spinae, it is difficult to find any occasion other than the climbing of stairs or inclines in which the stomach muscles are firmly contracted during a normal day's activities. So, throughout the day the stomach muscles generally rest while the back muscles do most of the work. Through the years the back muscles have become relatively the strongest muscles in the body. As they become stronger they become shorter, thereby increasing the pressure on the posterior edges of the discs and on the sacroiliac ligaments. The stomach muscles are unable to counteract this increased pressure because their lack of use has made them so weak and flabby that they merely stretch out and accommodate the pressure rather than prevent it. In extreme cases the abdominal wall collapses as the rectus abdominis divaricates. This occurs in some multiparous women. Whatever the cause of the sagging abdominal wall, visceroptosis follows, and it leads to strain on the lumbosacral ligament. This in turn produces stretching of the anterior common ligament which becomes thickened and even ossified (Helfet and Lee, 1978). Eventually this physiological attempt to buttress the lumbar spine fails and severe lumbar lordosis develops.

IN SUMMARY

108.   Muscle fatigue is electromyographically different from muscle spasm and occurs with overuse from postural or occupational activities.

Muscular fatigue may be relieved by resting the muscle or by promoting the blood flow within it.

109. Muscle fatigue in the erectores spinae muscles follows repeated forward bending, especially when using the hands. The muscles act as a bowstring as they hyperextend the lumbar spine.

110. Hyperextension of the spine is painful in some patients with pre-existing disc disease because nerve root compression is increased. A third source of pain arises from the spinal ligaments which are continuously stretched posterior to the vertebral bodies in the thoracolumbar junction and anterior to the vertebral bodies in the lumbar region. Bending forwards also strains the sacrospinous, sacrotuberous and anterior sacroiliac ligaments which prevent the sacrum from rotating forwards between the two halves of the pelvis.

111. Hyperextension can also occur in the sitting position and ligamentous stretching may give rise to pain. In most situations it is difficult to discern whether pain originates from posterior muscles or from ligaments.

112. The abdominal muscles are the antagonists of the erectores spinae and straighten the lumbar spine by pulling up on the front of the pelvis. Often the abdominal muscles are weak in contrast to the paraspinal muscles which are extremely strong.

113. The erectores spinae muscles shorten as they strengthen. The anterior sacroiliac ligaments thicken but finally fail and severe lumbar lordosis results.

CONCLUSION

The foregoing chapters have described progressions from one diseased state to another passing through various intermediate conditions. Variations in the order of the conditions in the sequences are common but two familiar examples are:

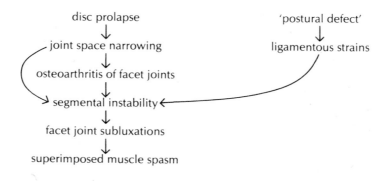

At any point in the chains, low back pain symptoms may be experienced but there is considerable overlap between the clinical features of the various stages. The most general diagnostic guide which encompasses the majority of back pain sufferers is:

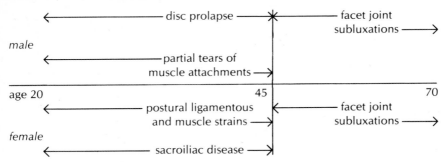

Of course there are many other possibilities – disc disease can occur in women and there are other pathologies which exist in the over 45-year-old age group. Nevertheless the four-stage classification not only fits well with the flexibility of the lumbar spine:

male	rigid		stiff	
	age 20	45	70	
female	lax		stiff	

but also with the rationale for treatment:

male	bed rest and epidural injections; analgesia		spinal manipulation; analgesia	
	age 20	45		70
female	exercise; posture correction; analgesia		spinal manipulation; analgesia	

Part 3
Conservative Treatment of the Abnormal Back

21 Bed rest, psychoactive drugs and epidural injections

Acute backs can be the result of new disease entities (such as prolapsed intervertebral discs or muscle tears), or exacerbations of existing conditions (such as facet joint subluxations secondary to segmental instability or long-standing disc disease). The latter, acute on chronic syndromes, are the more common especially in those patients older than 45 years. Patients younger than this tend to get prolapsed discs (if they are male) or strained ligaments (if they are female). Acute prolapsed discs are accompanied by agonizing pain and intense muscle spasm. Straight leg raising is nearly always reduced. These patients should be put to bed to rest, a treatment that is often prescribed for other causes of acute backs but is seldom necessary. Macnab (1977) points out that theoretical treatment must be tempered by reason. What about tomorrow's surgery for the dentist with an acute back pain? The experience of the lay world is that the majority of patients will get better just creeping around with their pain mollified by analgesics. Cyriax (1969) writes that getting out of bed will not increase the size of the disc protrusion, but merely cause additional pain. It is for the patient to decide which he dislikes more – not doing what he wants or getting increased pain if he does: 'There is no point, therefore, in keeping a patient of this sort in bed any longer than he wishes'.

If the pain is severe and the patient has to stay in bed, he should rest on a non-sagging but comfortable surface such as a firm mattress supported by a rigid board. The patient is advised to lie on his back with the knees propped up on pillows and with a pillow under the head. This position should be maintained as much of the time as possible.

If this position becomes too uncomfortable, the patient should turn on one side and draw up the knees, supporting the loin by a pillow to prevent the lumbar spine from sagging between the pillars of the shoulders and pelvis. If the duration of rest is prolonged, static leg exercises should be performed to prevent venous thrombosis. Using a bedpan at home is impractical but the use of crutches makes it easier for the patient to get to the bathroom. Pelvic traction in the acute disc prolapse can be applied by using a harness on an inclined bed. Three or four days spent thus can be more effective than much longer periods of bedrest and enable the individual with a large disc prolapse to reduce some of it and then be treated ambulant with support. In general, lumbar traction, either intermittent or continuous, appears to help some patients but the results are unpredictable. Traction should be given only if radiographs show no sign of a destructive lesion or subluxation.

Rest can be prescribed in an alternative form by confining the patient to a plaster jacket. Some time ago there was a vogue for the use of these jackets in the treatment of acute, incapacitating backache. Macnab (1977) believes that if the patient cannot work wearing a body jacket, he is better off in bed. Jackets, however, can be prescribed for patients who cannot take any time off work as long as the patient is able both to work and travel to work wearing the jacket. Macnab continues: 'while the jacket is being applied, an attempt must be made to flatten the lumbar spine. This can be achieved by having the patient stand with one foot on a stool. The plaster must be moulded so it presses into the abdomen, and by increasing abdominal pressure, unweights the spine' (Figure **21.1**).

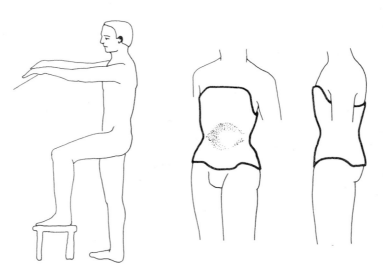

Figure 21.1   When a plaster body jacket is applied for the treatment of low back pain, the lumbar spine should be flattened by making the patient stand with one foot on a stool. The front of the cast should press firmly against the abdomen to increase intra-abdominal pressure and thereby 'unweight' the spine (from Macnab, 1977)

Cyriax (1969) suggests that a plaster jacket may be worn for a few days until a more suitable appliance is ready. Since a plaster cannot be made really tight or the patient's breathing will be restricted after meals, it should be abandoned as soon as an alternative is found. Macnab also believes there is no point in keeping the plaster jacket on for more than 1 week or 10 days. If the patient is still grossly incapacitated at the end of this time, the jacket should be removed and the patient should be sent to bed. If the pain has abated somewhat, the plaster should be bivalved and over the next 3 weeks worn during the day, while at work, being held in position by webbing straps. Cyriax's replacement appliance is the plastic jacket which weighs only one-quarter the weight of a plaster jacket. The plastic jacket can be worn for an indefinite period as it is taken off at night and can be tightened to fit as required.

In less severe cases a lumbar spinal corset with steel supports may suffice. Cyriax recommends that the two steels should be accurately moulded to the lumbar curve to maintain lordosis and to hold steady the joints 'in a good posture'. Macnab's advice is contrary and seems more reasonable. He writes that the most important component of a spinal brace is the abdominal binder which both pushes the centre of gravity of the patient backwards nearer the spine and enables the abdominal pressure to rise more easily thus providing hydrostatic support to the spine. Obese patients achieve the greatest benefit from the provision of a corset because obesity itself pulls the centre of gravity forward and causes the spine to hyperextend – reactions that are countered by an abdominal binder *as long as it is worn very tightly*. For this reason posterior steels in braces should not be bent to fit the lordotic curve as this loses an important function of the brace. Even when fitted accurately, corsets allow a considerable amount of spinal movement but they do act as postural educators by becoming uncomfortable when the patient bends too far forwards. Jayson (1978) does not encourage prolonged use of a corset for he writes that this can lead to spinal stiffness and weakness of paraspinal muscles. Cyriax allays this fear by explaining that these muscles extend as far as the neck and must still work to maintain the thorax erect.

Macnab believes that although analgesics are rarely needed once the patient is in bed, in the majority sedatives are essential. Jenkins, Ebbutt, and Evans (1976) compared the antidepressant imipramine with placebo in patients suffering from low back pain, because they had the impression that amongst the group of patients suffering from low backache a proportion are depressed. The purpose of the trial was to see whether it was possible to identify that group of patients and whether they would benefit from treatment with antidepressants. Over the whole sample there was no significant benefit as regards physical measurements or subjective assessments for imipramine over placebo. Analysis according to initial diagnosis showed nothing conclusive. Numerically, however, the use of imipramine produced a marked improvement in pain and stiffness in patients with 'disc lesion only' diagnosis, whereas placebo produced no improvement. This observation, although far from reaching statistical significance, suggested that some patients with acute disc prolapse do benefit from antidepressants.

Hingorani (1966) compared diazepam with placebo in a double-blind trial because he felt its muscle-relaxing properties might be of help to patients with lumbar spondylosis and prolapsed intervertebral discs. The patients were admitted to hospital and the medications were given firstly by injection for 1 day and then orally for 5 days. Both on subjective and objective grounds the results of the two treatments were comparable; thus at the dosage of diazepam used there was no evidence that it was superior to placebo.

Therefore, with antidepressants showing only a non-significant advantage, and with diazepam showing no advantage over placebo, are there any treatments that improve upon bedrest alone? Coomes (1961) compared bedrest with caudal epidural anaesthesia in outpatients with sciatica and found that the epidural group almost uniformly did much better than the bedrest group. Patients in the epidural group were up and about at a significantly earlier date and showed greater improvement in neurological signs. All of the patients started with nerve root pressure with neurological signs in the affected leg, and Coomes inferred that they were suffering from degenerative disease of the intervertebral discs. Lumbar disc disease was also the criterion of entry into the trial of Dilke, Burry, and Grahame (1973) when they examined the effect of extradural corticosteroid injections in patients with nerve root compression syndromes. Here 100 consecutive inpatients were assigned by random allocation to treatment and control groups. The control group received a superficial injection of normal saline into the interspinous ligament, whereas the treatment group received methylprednisolone in normal saline, administered into the extradural space by the lumbar route. Assessment during admission and after 3 months revealed statistically highly significant differences in respect of relief of pain and resumption of normal occupation in favour of the group treated by extradural injection.

Yates (1978) commented that despite the fact that it is generally agreed that not infrequently epidural injections produce dramatic relief of symptoms, there are differences of opinion on the indications, the route, the constituents and the volume. His crossover trial showed that the greatest improvement was noted after those injections containing steroid, suggesting that the action of a successful epidural injection is primarily anti-inflammatory and to a lesser extent hydrodynamic. This accorded with the previous findings of Beliveau (1971) and Sayle-Creer and Swerdlow (1969), although adhesions around the nerve roots can possibly be separated by this technique especially where fluid volumes of 100 ml or more are employed. Yates used the caudal route as do many other investigators. Advocates of both the caudal route and the lumbar route discuss the advantages and disadvantages of each at length, but the only controlled comparison of the two routes of injection is the trial of Sayle-Creer and Swerdlow which showed the two routes to be equally effective.

The indication for epidural injection should be a prolapsed intervertebral disc in the acute stage. I have made the mistake of attempting to undertake a trial of epidural anaesthesia in non-specific low back pain only to end up with extremely poor results. Acute disc prolapses are relatively uncommon and it is only in this indication that the injection is useful. Sayle-Creer and Swerdlow noted much higher success rates in acute cases and in those patients thought to be typical of presenting with disc lesions. The technique of the injection is described well by both Cyriax (1969) and Sharma (1977). Although it is usually regarded as a very safe procedure, infection has been reported, and Dougherty and Fraser (1978) question the use of intraspinal steroids in the treatment of disc-related sciatica.

IN SUMMARY

114. Acute backs can be the result of new disease entities (such as prolapsed intervertebral discs) or exacerbations of existing conditions (such as facet joint subluxations secondary to previous mechanical derangement).

115. The latter, acute on chronic syndromes, are the more common. Although bedrest is often prescribed for these patients it is seldom necessary.

116. Acute prolapsed intervertebral discs should be treated initially by bedrest but this should not be enforced if the patient wishes otherwise. Plaster jackets may be used as an alternative to bedrest for up to a week or so. In less severe cases, corsets may be worn provided they have a tight abdominal binder. Plastic jackets, which can be worn with less discomfort, are also available.

117. Antidepressants may be of help to some patients with acute disc prolapse. A controlled trial failed to show superiority of a muscle relaxant (diazepam) over placebo.

118. Controlled trials have shown epidural anaesthesia to be significantly better than both bedrest and a control injection in nerve root pressure syndromes. Other trials have shown steroid to be the important constituent of the injection, but the caudal and lumbar routes of injection appear to be equally effective. The injection should only be given in cases of acute disc prolapse and the aseptic technique should be impeccable.

22 Analgesics, acupuncture and TENS

Despite the large number of anti-inflammatory analgesic drugs available and the widespread prevalence of low back pain, controlled trials of medicines in the alleviation of this symptom are few. Yet in most instances rest and simple drugs are prescribed to those persons with back pain who consult their general practitioner (Working Group on Back Pain, 1979). The trials that do exist usually compare two drugs at a time. In the late 1960s and early 1970s one of these drugs was invariably indomethacin. The dose most often chosen was 75 mg per day in three divided doses. Jacobs and Grayson (1968) attempted to use 100 mg daily, but it became apparent that headache and nausea were troublesome so they reduced the dosage for subsequent patients to 75 mg daily for 2 days before using the larger dose of 100 mg for the next 5 days. They showed that indomethacin was significantly more effective than placebo in those patients with nerve root pain. On the other hand no difference was found between the treatments in the patients with uncomplicated low back pain. They postulated that the anti-inflammatory effect of indomethacin reduces inflammation around the nerve root in those suffering from radicular pain but in non-specific lesions they were dealing with a ligamentous lesion with no inflammation. In these latter cases the investigators advocated the use of an analgesic drug.

In the same year Goldie (1968) compared indomethacin with placebo in patients with an acute attack of sciatica because he too believed that an inflammatory reaction interfered with the nerve root. However, in his trial he was unable to show any advantage of indomethacin over placebo. Hingorani and Biswas (1970) compared oxyphenbutazone, a naturally occurring metabolite of phenylbutazone, with indomethacin but paracetamol was allowed as rescue analgesia to both drugs. He found more rapid pain relief with oxyphenbutazone but by day 7 its effect was equalled

Table 22.1 Drug trials in low back pain

Trial	Patients	Pain	Treatments	Control	Duration of Rx	Results
Goldie (1968)	inpatients	Low back pain with sciatic radiation; acute (<3 weeks)	indomethacin 75 mg daily. placebo	double-blind	2 weeks	no difference between indomethacin and placebo at 7 and 14 days
Jacobs and Grayson (1968)	outpatients	acute or acute-on-chronic lumbar pain	indomethacin 75–100 mg daily. placebo	double-blind, sequential	1 week	if nerve root pain indomethacin superior to placebo. If uncomplicated low back pain no difference between drugs
Hingorani and Biswas (1970)	inpatients	acute or acute-on-chronic low back pain	oxyphenbutazone 400 mg daily. indomethacin 100 mg daily, both plus paracetamol	double-blind	1 week	more rapid pain relief with oxyphenbutazone but equal by day 7
Hingorani (1971)	inpatients	acute or acute-on-chronic low back pain	{orphenadrine 210 mg daily paracetamol 2700 mg daily aspirin 1800 mg daily	double-blind	1 week	pain scores same with both drugs; forward flexion better with combination
Jaffé (1974)	outpatients	low back pain ± sciatica; two strata, acute or chronic	alclofenac 3 g daily indomethacin 150 mg daily	double-blind	1 week	two treatments equally effective; more erratic response by acute group
Hingorani and Templeton (1975)	inpatients	acute backache	azapropazone 1200 mg daily ketoprofen 200 mg daily, both plus paracetamol	double-blind, crossover	1 + 1 (placebo) + 1 week	more patients preferred third week's treatment. No more paracetamol usage in second (placebo) week
Grevsten and Johannson (1975)	outpatients	acute or acute-on-chronic backache ± sciatica; paired patients	phenylbutazone 600→ 300 mg daily. placebo	double-blind	2 weeks	improvement (often in 2–4 days) in 88 per cent phenylbutazone and 47 per cent placebo patients (significant difference)
Ciocci (1976)	outpatients	1. acute lumbago 2. chronic lumbago 3. sciatica 4. spondylarthritis	indomethacin 75–200 mg daily	open	2–4 weeks	good results in 1. 52 per cent 2. 90 per cent 3. 50 per cent 4. 78 per cent

by that of indomethacin. Paracetamol consumption did not differ significantly between the two groups and there was no difference in tenderness.

Grevsten and Johannson (1975) compared phenylbutazone to placebo and found an improvement in symptoms (often within 2—4 days of starting) in 88 per cent of the patients who received phenylbutazone and in 47 per cent of the patients who received placebo. This difference is significant at the 5 per cent level. They believed that phenylbutazone worked by suppression of the non-specific inflammatory reaction with oedema which occurs on straining of ligaments, intervertebral discs or intervertebral joints: 'The underlying mechanism of the pain in acute lumbagoischias is not properly understood but the inflammatory oedema probably irritates the nerves in the outer layer of the annulus fibrosus, in the longitudinal ligaments and in the capsular tissue of the intervertebral joints'.

These trials are summarised in Table 22.1 together with others comparing less widely used medicines. The trial by Ciocci (1976), although an open trial, is included because it showed the better response to indomethacin of chronic (as opposed to acute) symptoms. This confirmed the impression of Jaffé (1974) who reported a more erratic response in those patients with acute low back pain. In acute or acute-on-chronic backache the placebo, indomethacin and phenylbutazone comparisons can be summarized:

indomethacin	equivalent to placebo
(75—100 mg daily)	
(except in nerve root pain then	
indomethacin superior to placebo)	
oxyphenbutazone	quicker acting than indomethacin
(400 mg daily)	(100 mg daily)
(but same at 1 week)	
phenylbutazone	significantly superior to placebo
(600 mg falling to 300 mg daily)	

Because of the difficulty of equating results between trials of different design, we (Evans, Burke, and Newcombe, 1980) chose to examine the marketed formulations of six treatments in patients suffering from acute exacerbations of low back pain using a single-blind trial of three-period, crossover design. We studied 60 ambulant outpatients who complained of acute-on-chronic low back pain. The presence of sciatica or femoral root pain in addition to lumbar pain was no bar to selection. Each patient was allocated according to a random list to a treatment sequence of three drugs which were administered consecutively for 1 week each. No other analgesic or anti-inflammatory medication was permitted during the 3 treatment weeks.

The patient's estimation of pain according to the scale 0 = nil, 1 = mild, 2 = moderate, 3 = severe was recorded daily on a diary card. The cards also contained daily records of numbers of capsules or tablets taken, reason for incomplete compliance if appropriate and other symptoms or events. After 3 weeks the patient expressed an opinion for the best treatment of the three he or she received and the worst. The six drugs were administered in maximal recommended dosages and were coded:

A	aspirin	3600 mg daily
B	{ dextropropoxyphene plus { paracetamol	{ 260 mg daily { 2600 mg daily
C	indomethacin	150 mg daily
D	mefenamic acid	1500 mg daily
E	paracetamol	4000 mg daily
F	phenylbutazone	300 mg daily

Of the 60 patients 40 were female. The mean age (±s.d.) was 47.0 (±9.2) years. The age structures and sex ratios were similar in the subgroups of patients receiving each medicine.

There was no evidence that spinal anterior flexion altered significantly during the course of the treatment period, nor that its rate of change was related to the degree of mobility of the patient at the start of the trial.

In the following tables (Tables 22.2 to 22.5) the mean values for each of the responses are serially ordered from the best to the worst. Pain index was summated over the 6 non-clinic days on a particular treatment. Average daily pain indices are shown in Table 22.2.

Table 22.2   Mean daily pain index and ranking order of trial medications

Medication	D	A	F	C	E	B
Mean daily pain index	1.375	1.425	1.433	1.487	1.660	1.713

$p < 0.05$ (spanning D to E)
$p < 0.05$ (spanning A to B)

Differences between the six treatments were significant ($p < 0.05$): according to the Duncan test (1955), D (mefenamic acid) was preferable to E (paracetamol) and B (dextropropoxyphene plus paracetamol), and A (aspirin) was preferable to B. D was the most effective drug for reducing pain but detailed examination of the results showed that this did not apply if the pain was brought on by sneezing. In that case A and F (phenylbutazone) did comparatively well. In terms of interaction with the binary term radiating or not-radiating, D performed extremely well in pain which radiated and in this respect differed from F and C (indomethacin).

As we are treating a symptom in low back pain, not a disease, it is important to identify the kind of patient for whom a particular treatment is preferable. Pain brought on by sneezing is usually regarded as being indicative of nerve root compression. In this symptom the anti-inflammatory drugs aspirin and phenylbutazone do comparatively well possibly, as Grevsten and Johannson (1975) postulated, by reducing the inflammatory oedema which was irritative to the nerve roots. Other pains, irrespective of whether they radiate or not, have been attributed to various tissues including ligaments and the capsular tissue of the intervertebral joints. Here a strong analgesic effect (as provided by mefenamic acid) seems preferable to an anti-inflammatory effect (as provided by phenylbutazone and indomethacin). The poor performance of indomethacin in our trial agreed with the findings of Goldie (1968) but was at variance with those of Jacobs and Grayson (1968) (where indomethacin was superior to placebo in those patients with nerve root pain, agreeing with the concept of using anti-inflammatory agents when there is pressure on the nerve roots).

The number of tablets or capsules taken were summated over the 6 non-clinic days in each treatment week. The results are the percentages of the recommended doses that the patient reported having taken. The differences between treatments were large and significant (Table 22.3).

Table 22.3   Percentage of recommended dose of trial medications taken by patients and ranking order

Medication	F	D	E	A	C	B
Per cent recommended dose	96.5	91.8	89.8	80.2	76.2	71.7

$p < 0.05$
$p < 0.01$
$p < 0.01$
$p < 0.05$
$p < 0.01$
$p < 0.05$

Table 22.4   Number of defaults in treatment and ranking order of trial medication

Medication	F	D	E	A	C	B
Maximum number defaults possible	30	30	30	30	30	30
Total number defaults observed	6	8	9	13	14	17

A patient was said to default from the full regimen for a particular treatment if he took fewer than the prescribed number of tablets on any of the 6 non-clinic days for which that treatment was prescribed (Table 22.4).

The total defaults were not spread evenly over the six treatments ($\chi^2 = 12.39$, $df = 5$, $p < 0.05$). If we restrict attention to defaults due partly or entirely to side-effects, the advantage of D, E and F becomes much more marked ($\chi^2 = 29.48$, $p < 0.001$). These latter three treatments were much more acceptable and they contained a higher proportion of patients with no

Table 22.5   Patients' preference of trial medications

Medication	F	D	C	B	E	A
Mean rank	1.68	1.75	1.98	2.07	2.15	2.37

$\longmapsto \qquad\qquad p<0.05 \qquad\qquad \longmapsto$

side-effects at all. The proportions with neurological side-effects were higher on A, B and C.

For a patient's preference, ranks of 1, 2 and 3 were used to denote the best, middle and worst of the three treatments. The stated preferences were not affected materially by recall bias, since the mean ranks for the first, second and third treatments administered in order were 2.03, 2.08 and 1.88 which did not differ significantly. Mean ranks for the medications are shown in Table 22.5.

Significant differences existed between treatments, and an adaptation of Duncan's test shows F and D superior to A at the 5 per cent significance level. We asked patients if they thought they had received each medicine before and analysed preferences separately for 'previous exposure' and 'no previous exposure'. In general, a drug performed slightly worse if it was recognized although the difference was not significant.

The statistical interpretation of this trial showed consistently superior performances by mefenamic acid (D) and phenylbutazone (F) with little to choose between the two. Mefenamic acid was best on 'any side-effects' and on pain index, and came a close second to phenylbutazone in terms of overall preference, spinal anterior flexion, tablets taken, total defaults and defaults attributed to side-effects. They were joint best for neurological and gastrointestinal side-effects. All things considered, whichever the patient prefers of mefenamic acid or phenylbutazone would be the treatment of choice.

Despite the absence of serious side-effects in this small sample, a medical interpretation must take account of rare, but potentially dangerous, events. Mefenamic acid rarely causes a Coombs-positive haemolytic anaemia (Scott, Myles, and Bacon, 1968) whereas phenylbutazone can cause blood dyscrasias. Hart (1978) writes that although highly effective, it is wise to use phenylbutazone only where a less potentially dangerous agent fails to control symptoms.

We tested our pain scores for any relationship there might be with age (less than 45 years, 45 years and over). The total pain scores were slightly higher in the older group but there was a significant reduction in pain over the 3 weeks. This was similar in both age groups. Therefore anti-inflammatory analgesics, particularly mefenamic acid and phenylbutazone, are important treatments in all four quadrants of our sex/age diagram.

When Mendelson et al. (1977) reviewed clinical studies in the use of acupuncture for the relief of chronic pain, they found that less than half of the 21 studies included a control group. Yet this treatment technique would seem to lend itself readily to controlled studies by the use of sham acupuncture, that is needles randomly placed in areas not considered to have any bearing on the patient's pain. However Mark (1973) believes that double-blind studies of acupuncture are not feasible because the correct placement of acupuncture needles requires cooperation of the patient in reporting paraesthesiae, a sensation of soreness or mild discomfort, and hence renders useless efforts to deceive him with placebo needles deliberately inserted elsewhere.

Edelist, Gross, and Langer (1976) did not subscribe to this objection when they studied 30 patients who had failed to get relief from their low back pain with conventional therapy (and were thought to be suffering from intervertebral disc disease). They assigned 15 patients randomly to a treatment group who received true acupuncture on three occasions at 2-day intervals, whereas the other 15 underwent sham acupuncture with the same number of needles but placed in areas in the back and legs where there are no classical acupuncture points. Their observer was unaware of the treatment group the patient had been in when he placed them into one of two categories – no improvement and significant improvement. There was no significant difference between the true acupuncture (46 per cent improvement) and sham acupuncture (40 per cent improvement) groups.

These authors used the acupuncture points Ta-ch'ang-ÿu bilaterally and Ch'êng-san bilaterally. Ta-ch'ang-ÿu is 3.6 cm lateral to the midline at a level between the fourth and fifth lumbar vertebrae. Ch'êng-san is at the distal margin of the gastrocnemious muscle, between its medial and lateral heads. These were the acupuncture points the authors discovered being used in the People's Republic of China. When Mendelson et al. (1977) circulated a questionnaire to 50 members of the Australian Medical Acupuncture Society, the treatment methods currently in use for the relief of chronic low back pain showed a surprisingly large variation in the techniques used. Many of the respondents referred to the need to vary the technique to suit the patient without, however, being more specific. After the poor results in the study by Edelist, Gross, and Langer (1976) the authors write that their acupuncturist may not have been as skilled as acupuncturists reporting better results. This factor is difficult to evaluate but my preference must lie with the one who was prepared to examine his treatment in a controlled manner.

Laitinen (1976) compared acupuncture with transcutaneous electric nerve stimulation (TENS) in the treatment of 100 patients with sacrolumbalgia or ischialgia of more than 6 months' duration. The patients received one of the two treatments two to ten times at weekly intervals, each treatment lasting for 20 minutes. The same bilateral stimulation points (two on each side) were used for the 50 patients treated with acupuncture as for the 50 patients treated with TENS. There were no statistical differences between the responses to the two treatments. Satisfactory responses were found more frequently in the acupuncture group than in the TENS group both in the short-term (58 per cent to 46 per cent) and 6 months after treatment (33 per cent to 21 per cent). These ratios were similar to that found by Fox and Melzack (1976) when they compared acupuncture with TENS in the treatment of chronic low back pain. Twelve patients received both acupuncture and TENS with the treatment orders balanced. Pain relief greater than 33 per cent was produced in 75 per cent of the patients by acupuncture, and in 66 per cent by electrical stimulation. The mean duration of pain relief was 40 hours after acupuncture and 23 hours after electrical stimulation. Although the mean scores are larger for acupuncture than for transcutaneous stimulation, statistical analyses of the data failed to reveal significant differences between the two treatments on any of the measures. The patients received both treatments twice and in every case there was 1 week between any one treatment and the next. Acupuncture was carried out by the insertion of a needle into points B24, B26, and B62 on the bladder meridian – points which are commonly used for the treatment of backache – with strong manual rotation for one minute at each successive point (Figure **22.1**). TENS was carried out by means of a disc electrode applied for 10 min at each of the same points in succession, with an indifferent electrode placed at a distant site.

Melzack (1973) suggests that acupuncture and transcutaneous electrical stimulation both fall into the category of 'hyperstimulation analgesia' and are simply methods of producing brief pain to relieve chronic, intense pain. Intense peripheral stimulation would produce a predominantly small fibre input which gives rise to pain but would also activate brain stem inhibitory fibres which in turn block pain signals from other areas. The fact that many patients reported that their pain was still diminished 4 months after termination of the treatment is of interest. TENS and acupuncture, however, are not cures and repeated treatments are usually necessary to provide continuing periods of relief.

In a later work, Melzack (1975) stimulated three kinds of sites with TENS – trigger zones (using palpation for painful area or the maps of Travell and Rinzler, 1952), peripheral nerve roots and acupuncture points. There is a high degree of correlation between trigger zones and acupuncture points designated for the same pain patterns; moreover these points frequently lie over a major sensory nerve. Low back pain and sciatica are frequently associated with a trigger point on the buttock which lies over the sciatic nerve and a major acupuncture point designated for this type of pain also lies at the same site. The average pain decrease during stimulation sessions was 75 per cent for pain due to peripheral nerve injury, 66 per cent for phantom limb pain, 62 per cent for shoulder-arm pain and 60 per cent for low back pain.

These workers all used high frequency electrical stimulation in trains of

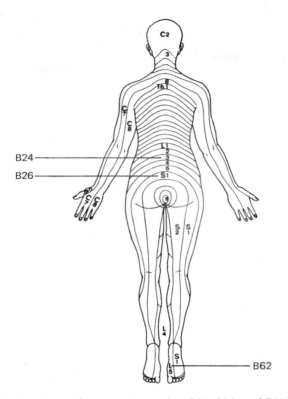

Figure 22.1 Locations of acupuncture points B24, B26, and B62 on the bladder meridian (from Fox and Melzack, 1976)

approximately 60 cycles/sec. Andersson *et al.* (1976) evaluated the pain-suppressive effect of different frequencies in 12 patients with severe, chronic pain in the back and/or the legs. The patients received sessions of both low frequency stimulation (2 cycles/sec) and high frequency stimulation (50–100 cycles per sec). The low frequency stimulation induced a partial pain relief in only one patient whereas stimulation with high frequency gave a suppression of pain in seven patients. The effect of high frequency stimulation on the pain was quite different as compared to that of a frequency of 2 cycles/sec. With the former, a marked pain relief was achieved within a few minutes when stimulation was applied to the painful areas or to areas overlying nerves innervating the regions of pain. The effect was shortlasting in most cases and the pain started to increase, usually within 30 min. The reproducibility of the pain-relieving effects was good. Any cumulative tendencies such as increasing pain suppression or more long-lasting effects were not observed, neither was there any lasting pain relief in any patient. No serious adverse effects of either low or high frequency stimulation were reported, neither did the physical re-examination disclose any impairment or improvement of the neuro-orthopaedic status. The authors concluded that the pain suppression is not due to a mere psychological distraction or suggestion but implies a basic neurophysiological mechanism.

Wilber (1975) describes a novel variation of acupuncture – sedation of the active acupuncture loci by means of one to six injections of a local anaesthetic/cortisone combination at weekly intervals. He describes the treatment of 23 patients suffering from low back pain with no obvious medical or surgical disease. Subcutaneously into each active acupuncture locus were injected 1 ml of a combination of equal parts of 1 per cent xylocaine and methylprednisolone. His trial was uncontrolled so success rates cannot be compared with the placebo response, nevertheless he commonly found active acupuncture loci in patients with 'facet syndrome', back pain secondary to trauma and chronic back pain. He rarely found active acupuncture loci in patients with acute herniated nucleus pulposus, neurogenic disorders, back pain associated with abdominal disorders and psychogenic back pain. Bourne (1979) also found less good results where demonstrable radiological intervertebral disc lesions were present (40 per cent failures as opposed to 20 per cent failures) when he injected the point of maximum tenderness with a combination of 1 ml of 2 per cent xylocaine and 1 ml of triamcinolone acetonide. He describes the treatment of 115 patients suffering from chronic backache by injections sometimes down to the level of the deep fascia in locations determined by a bracketing technique.

The role of acupuncture and TENS in the treatment of low back pain has yet to be determined. It is possible that acupuncture and high frequency electrical stimulation will turn out to be useful in the alleviation of pain in the short-term. Local anaesthetic injections into the subcutaneous tissues may also prove to be efficacious in low back pain which is not due to intervertebral disc lesions.

IN SUMMARY

119.   Despite the large number of anti-inflammatory analgesic drugs available and the widespread prevalence of low back pain, controlled trials of medicines in the alleviation of this symptom are few.

120.   Where a nerve root lesion is believed responsible for symptoms, it is postulated that there is inflammation around the nerve root which can be relieved by anti-inflammatory agents. There is confirmatory evidence that phenylbutazone, and to a lesser extent indomethacin, are effective in this situation.

121.   Where low back pain is thought to be due to a non-specific lesion (perhaps a ligamentous lesion or one in the capsular tissue of inter-

vertebral joints) an analgesic drug is proposed. There is confirmatory evidence that mefenamic acid is effective in this situation.

122. Overall, phenylbutazone and mefenamic acid are the drugs of choice in the treatment of low back pain, with little to choose between the two. Pain reduction is similar in those patients aged less than or greater than 45 years of age.

123. Despite the great variation in acupuncture techiques between individual practitioners treating low back pain, there is no evidence that the response to true acupuncture is superior to the response to sham acupuncture.

124. There is no evidence that the response to acupuncture differs from that due to transcutaneous electric nerve stimulation (TENS) in the treatment of low back pain.

125. There is some evidence that the response to high frequency TENS (50–100 cycles/sec) is superior to the response to low frequency TENS (2 cycles/sec). The former has not been shown to have any cumulative effect or provide appreciable long-lasting benefit, whereas for the latter it is difficult to show any effect at all.

126. The classical acupuncture points were used in the studies quoted above for both true acupuncture and for TENS. These points correlate highly with the trigger zones described by Travell and Rinzler (1952) and frequently lie over a major sensory nerve.

127. Active acupuncture loci or points of maximum tenderness can be injected with a combination of a local anaesthetic and corticosteroid. Good results are claimed as long as the back pain is not due to intervertebral disc lesions.

23 Posture correction and exercise

Coplans (1978) defines man's ideal posture as that which can be maintained most effortlessly throughout the activities of daily living. Thus posture must be considered in relation to activities and not to man as a standing, motionless pillar. Nor must mechanically satisfactory posture be confused with appearance. There is no universal 'good posture', although when standing for prolonged periods the body weight should be supported primarily on the heels and the chest should be shifted slightly forward so a crease is formed across the upper abdomen (Williams, 1974). One or (preferably) both knees should be slightly bent or flexed.

With regard to the configuration of the lumbar spine, most workers have used different classifications from the dichotomy of static and dynamic lumbar spines proposed by Delmas (1974). Beck and Killus (1973) compared these various classifications but found little conformity (Figure **23.1**). Even those spines which in their opinion were highly pathological could be found in conformity with one of the posture types.

Beck and Killus developed a system of cartesian coordinates to measure spinal columns in two planes. The 150 spines they tested were distributed normally and they were able to show only one ideal type of spinal column in young men (Figure **23.2**). Hence, by the use of mathematical and statistical methods it was not possible to find evidence for the presence of several different constitutional posture types.

If a population is represented by a normal distribution of spinal shapes, deviation from the norm can take place in two directions. This leads on the one hand to the stiff, straight back epitomized by 'military bearing' and on the other to the hypermobile, sinuous back so often encountered in young persons. Although both deviations are prone to low back pain, it is the latter group which suffers from chronic lower ligamentous strain, often called

213

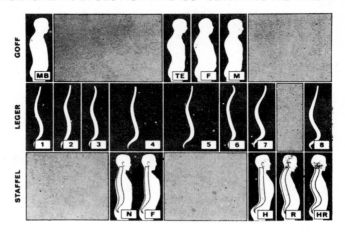

Figure 23.1   Classifications of postural types (from Beck and Killus, 1973)

postural backache. This is extremely common in young women and produces a nagging, low-grade ache which often persists for many years. The lumbar or lumbosacral aching is worse on prolonged standing, especially if combined with leaning forwards or aggravated by the wearing of high-heeled shoes. Wyke (1976) postulates that the pain is produced from the ligaments and their aponeuroses when these tissues are subjected to abnormal mechanical stresses by prolonged standing or by persistently distorted postures often in occupational circumstances.

The common mechanical derangement is a forward inclination of the pelvis which in turn necessitates hyperextension of the lumbar spine in order to maintain an upright position. This results in abnormal strain on ligaments, interspinal joints and the supporting musculature. The basic cause of the downward sagging of the front of the pelvis appears to be due to weakness of the abdominal muscles which form the anterior portion of the cylinder wall of the trunk. Treatment must aim for good abdominal musculature to sustain intra-abdominal pressure and to prevent the forward pelvic tilting and resultant exaggerated lordosis. This objective is opposite to that of the traditional exercises commonly prescribed to patients with back pain which set out to strengthen the paraspinal muscles. Nachemson (1976) does not know of any evidence that subjects with low back pain possess particularly weak muscles. On the other hand, he says it is known that in certain situations, for example when lifting and carrying heavy objects, the increase of intra-abdominal and intrathoracic pressure, from contraction of abdominal and costal muscles, will help relieve some of the load of the lumbar spine. He, therefore, regards it as rational that patients who are in a rehabilitation programme after a long period of low back pain should perform isometric abdominal muscle exercises. Also in these subjects, special reference should be given to the training of the quadriceps muscles,

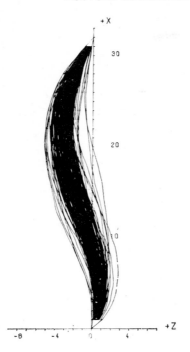

Figure 23.2   Computer plotting of 150 spines (from Beck and Killus, 1973)

as they take more load when lifting weights the correct way than the incorrect way. When lifting weights it is generally accepted that the patient should be instructed to flex the knees and keep the spine as straight as possible, so making use of the knee extensors to do the lifting, not the back extensors. Furthermore Dehlin *et al.* (1978) found that a group of nursing aides with lumbar spine symptoms had significantly lower quadriceps muscle strength compared to a group without back symptoms, whereas their trunk muscle strength was similar.

Not only are back extension exercises unnecessary, but many of these exercises increase the load on the lumbar spine to such an extent that it reaches magnitudes as high as those measured in standing and leaning forward with weights in the hands – one of the worst activities for patients with back trouble. As far as disc pressure is concerned, isometrically performed exercises seem less dangerous. Even among practitioners who attribute the majority of back pain to disc degenerative changes causing narrowing of the neural foramina, there are those like Williams (1974) who believe that symptoms are exacerbated by increased lordosis and they advocate the strengthening of abdominal musculature. Coplans (1978) agrees with the importance of abdominal strengthening exercises but adds that synchronized respiration plays an important part. The patient is taught to contract the abdominal wall and at the same time perform strong exhalation.

Isometric flexion exercises have been shown experimentally by Kendall and Jenkins (1968) to be significantly superior to the exercises frequently recommended 'to strengthen and mobilize the spine'. They compared the best known 'back extension exercises' with both 'mobilizing exercises' and a group of exercises that achieve their effect by 'isometric contraction of the abdominal muscles'. The latter exercises were

(1) lying on the back with the knees bent and contracting the abdominal and pelvic floor and hip adductor muscles; and
(2) standing whilst contracting abdominal and pelvic floor and hip adductor muscles.

The exercises were repeated 12 times, three times daily, and the standing position exercises were repeated as often as possible during the day. In a double-blind, controlled trial containing 47 patients, two stopped treatment because their backache was made worse by the exercises and they were both in the back extension exercise group. A statistically significantly larger group of patients benefited from the isometric abdominal muscle exercises than from either of the other two groups or both groups added together. Lidström and Zachrisson (1970) evaluated physical therapy in low back pain and sciatica and verified the uselessness of strengthening the back muscles. They showed that an increase in dorsal muscle strength was not accompanied by a decrease in pain. The treatment group that fared best in their study received a combination of intermittent traction of the lumbar spine and isometric training of the glutei and abdominal muscles.

To help in the maintenance of his ideal posture, Williams (1974) advocated the wearing of a shoe which necessitates a slightly forward bend of the trunk in order to keep the centre of gravity of the body within the base formed by the margins of the feet. This 'negative-heel' shoe, so called because the heel is the thinnest part of the sole, has been claimed to help low back pain sufferers but reports of experimental studies are lacking. In contrast, the extended-heel shoe has been shown to reduce significantly the degree of lumbar lordosis within 6 weeks of its use. This is any shoe or sandal with a backward heel extension which allows the wearer to lean backwards beyond the angle at which he or she would normally tip (Figure **23.3**).

Although a patient exercising in extended-heel sandals may appear to be undertaking back extension exercises, it is important to distinguish between the *active* back muscle exercises of the latter and the *passive* back extension seen in the sandal exercises. In this case the active exercises are those to the abdominal musculature and quadriceps femoris muscles (Evans, 1980).

Correction of posture and muscle strengthening by exercise are the only measures that are likely to reduce the recurrence of symptoms in the long-term. Isometric abdominal muscle exercises help a large number of sufferers

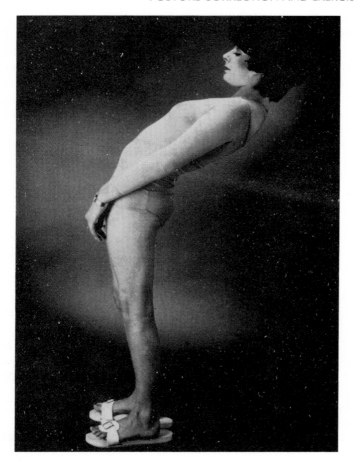

Figure 23.3 Patient exercising in extended-heel shoes

and the various exercise regimens are described well by Coplans (1978). Whether other patients might benefit from back *extension* exercises has yet to be demonstrated by controlled clinical trials. McKenzie (1979) examined the role of frequent *passive* extension movements (not unlike the extended-heel shoe exercises when in the standing position) on the prophylaxis in recurrent low back pain. His trial was uncontrolled and he was the first to state 'regardless of the type of treatment applied, approximately 80 per cent of all patients will be better at the end of two months'. Nevertheless it appeared that passive extension reduced the pain in the majority of his patients.

It is possible that McKenzie's patients came from the opposite end of the distribution curve from those benefiting from isometric abdominal exercises and they may represent divergence from the lumbar spinal norm in the other (towards a flat lumbar spine) direction. For example 87 per cent of his patients had a reduced lumbar lordosis and nearly all of these complained of back pain on prolonged sitting. In addition 61 per cent were males, 64 per cent were older than 40 years and 50 per cent had scoliosis. If there is only one lumbar spinal distribution for all patients perhaps the extremes of this can be corrected by abdominal exercises if the patient's spine is too lordotic, or paraspinal muscle exercises if the patient's spine is too flat. There is a need to extend the work of Beck and Killus (1973) to the spines of young women and to those of older patients of both sexes to determine normal lumbar shapes. Remaining hypothetical but reverting to the generalities outlined at the end of Part 2, we may find:

	<45 years	>45 years
♂	pain on sitting flat lumbar spine disc disease R$_x$ extension exercises	
♀	pain on standing lordotic lumbar spine ligamentous disease R$_x$ flexion exercises	

The young female quarter of this diagram has been established by the scientific method. Despite the evidence from the same sources disparaging the validity of the exercises proposed in the young male quarter, there might be a role for back-extension exercises in a select population group yet to be defined. This diagram is a generalization. Some male patients will have symptoms and signs typical of the female quarter and vice versa. In these paradoxical situations the treatment should be prescribed according to the symptoms and signs, not according to the patient's sex.

IN SUMMARY

128. There is only one ideal shape of lumbar spinal column for young men. This may be the ideal shape for women and old men as well but evidence is at present lacking. If there is one distribution of lumbar spinal shapes, deviation from the norm may take place in two directions.

129. Deviation to the more curved spine is common in young women and leads to low back pain originating from the ligaments. The mechanical derangement is a forward inclination of the pelvis which in turn necessitates hyperextension of the lumbar spine in order to maintain an upright posture. The basic cause is weakness of the abdominal

muscles which form the anterior portion of the cylinder wall of the trunk.

130. The abdominal musculature should be exercised isometrically by various well-described exercises or by exercising in extended-heel shoes.

131. Deviation to the flatter spine has been shown to be associated with low back pain which is helped by passive back extension procedures. The role of active back extension exercises has yet to be delineated but there is ample evidence that they should not be prescribed routinely to all low back pain sufferers.

24 Spinal manipulation

Spinal manipulation by its very name must involve manual treatment of the patient by the therapist, but the title unfortunately refers to many different forms of treatment. This chapter will deal only with manipulation without anaesthesia. In Britain spinal manipulation as practised by medically qualified practitioners usually entails a rotational thrust to the subcervical vertebral column whilst distraction is applied along its length. These are small-amplitude, high velocity movements going beyond the normal active ranges of motion. Mobilization techniques are repetitive gentle oscillatory movements within the normal active ranges of motion. These are usually practised by physiotherapists but are sometimes included under the umbrella title of spinal manipulation. Unless otherwise stated, manipulation in this chapter refers to rotational thrust with distraction. This basic technique has been the mainstay of whole disciplines of therapy usually practised by medically unqualified persons, but evidence is lacking for any effect beyond that provided by the basic manoeuvre. It is partly on account of the diversity of techniques and practitioners, and the lack of any critical review of their work, that this form of treatment has become one of the most emotive of subjects in modern medicine. Only recently has the orthodox medical fraternity accepted spinal manipulation as a valid form of treatment, although its history goes back thousands of years and has been reviewed excellently by Schiötz and Cyriax (1975).

Acceptance has followed controlled clinical trials which have started to delineate the indications for this mode of treatment. Glover, Morris and Khosla (1974) were the first to publish a clinical trial of rotational manipulation in low back pain. Their cases, all factory workers, included only those patients with pain on one side of the back so that there was a contralateral side for comparison. Most advocates of this procedure would invalidate this criterion as they would not consider it reasonable to manipulate one side of the spine only. Rotational manipulation twists the whole spine in the lumbar and thoracic regions and acts rather like a 'mechanical ECT' – specific manipulations to a single vertebra are not possible and thrusts in one direction only would seem a restriction serving no useful purpose. In this single-blind trial Glover, Morris and Khosla compared the effect of manipulation with that of detuned shortwave diathermy which acted as a placebo treatment. Although each of the two treatment groups showed progressive and marked improvement in pain relief during the 7-day trial period, there was no difference between the two except that immediately after treatment the relief from pain in the manipulated group was always greater than in the controls. Combining the two treatment groups showed that those with less than a week's history of back pain improved more rapidly than those with more than a week's history, but this difference was not statistically significant.

Coxhead (1974) completed a pilot study to assess the efficacy of the common forms of physiotherapy used in the treatment of sciatica with or without low back pain. Included among the nine treatments were the manipulations advocated by Maitland (1977) – earlier in this chapter described as mobilizations. The results of the main study are awaited keenly, but whatever the outcome interpretation will highlight the difficulty of comparing one type of manipulation with others. Diversity between methods was the biggest drawback of the multicentre trial by Doran and Newell (1975) which combined the results from several manipulators using different techniques. The various manipulations were compared collectively with physiotherapy, corsets and analgesic therapy. The criteria of entry excluded patients with symptoms of nerve root compression therefore limiting the trial to the mildest forms of back pain. Patients over the age of 50 years were also excluded – the significance of this omission will become apparent later. Although there was no significant difference between treatments at 3 weeks, proportionately more of the patients in the manipulation group reported improvement than patients in the other three groups. Correspondingly more manipulated patients failed to complete the 3-week treatment course because they were better. After 6 weeks there were no significant differences between treatments but so many additional treatments had been added to the original treatments that these and subsequent assessments were difficult to interpret. Nevertheless the investigators concluded that there was nothing to choose between the 'active' treatments but they were marginally better than analgesics. This was not unexpected because the analgesic (paracetamol) was prescribed to each of the three groups in addition to the 'active' treatment; thus the trial really amounted to the investigation of various 'active' treatments plus analgesics versus analgesics alone. At 3 months there were no significant differences between the treatment groups, but more of those treated with manipulation were 'completely relieved' than those treated with alternative therapies. Interestingly, for those treated with manipulation there was a strong correlation between the assessments at 6 weeks and at 3 months; in the other groups this strong positive correlation did not exist. The authors indicated that there is little point in continuing manipulation if there is no improvement after 3 weeks. At 1 year the results of the various treatments were even closer together.

Doran and Newell (1975) concluded that none of the methods showed any great superiority. Patients treated with analgesics alone fared marginally worse than those on the other three treatments. The corset was as effective as the other treatments in the long-term. Manipulation produced an early response in a few cases but nothing was found at the initial assessment to identify in advance the relatively small number of patients who benefited from manipulation.

Our trial (Evans et al., 1978) was set up specifically to answer this last question. Several of the design features of the previously described trial were used, but a smaller number of patients were studied in great depth and they were all manipulated by *the same* medically qualified therapist using a rotational thrust with distraction both to the left and to the right. As Doran and Newell's trial showed excellent correlation between the results at 6 weeks and 3 months for those treated with manipulation, we restricted our trial to 6 weeks' duration and compared manipulation plus codeine phosphate to codeine phosphate alone. The results were consistent with those found in both the trials of Glover, Morris and Khosla and Doran and Newell, producing some important corroborations. For example, Glover et al. stratified their group of patients by number and duration of previous attacks. Their stratum resembling the patients in our trial behaved similarly in that during the first week after manipulation the manipulated group suffered more pain than the control group. By equating subjective assessments in the trials of Doran and Newell and Evans et al., very similar results were evident at 3 weeks in the groups receiving manipulative treatment.

Furthermore, in our trial there was a significant increase in spinal flexion measured clinically during the 3-week period of manipulation followed by a significant decrease in the 3-week period after manipulation. Although the first week of manipulative treatment was more painful than the corresponding week in the control group, in the second and third weeks there was less pain in the manipulated group. Pain scores were reduced to a significant degree within 4 weeks of starting manipulation. The most important contribution of this trial was the identification of those patients deriving most benefit from this form of treatment. The patients who deteriorated or remained unchanged (non-responders) were compared to those who markedly improved (responders). To increase the sensitivity between groups, patients who slightly improved were omitted from this comparison. The non-responders were significantly younger than the responders with a demarcation age of about 45 years. The median age of the responders was 50 years – half of these responders would have been excluded by the acceptance criterion of Doran and Newell's trial. The duration of back pain was longer in the non-responders in spite of the younger ages of the patients in that group. The age of onset was very significantly earlier in non-responders compared to responders. Radiographs of the spine and radiographic assessment of spinal motion were of no value in predicting or assessing the response of the patients to manipulation. In Part II of this trial (Roberts et al., 1978) we concluded that although radiography of the lumbar spine is a commonly requested investigation, it contributes little to the management of such patients except to exclude serious spinal pathology before any form of physical treatment is commenced.

Sims-Williams et al. (1978) reported on a controlled trial of mobilization and manipulation for patients with low back pain in general practice. Once again Maitland's techniques were employed, so the treatment was primarily mobilization. Patients were excluded if they were thought by the physiotherapist to be unlikely to benefit from mobilization – a feature of the methodology which seems to be anticipating the result and if used frequently must have added considerable bias to the trial. In addition, traction and exercises were included into the 'mobilization package' and the contribution of each modality of treatment is difficult to apportion. Nevertheless reduced pain at 1 month was more common in patients who had received active treatment than in the controls (who received a placebo therapy of microwave) but the difference was only of borderline significance. No change in spinal flexion had occurred in the active-treatment group but there was a significant decrease in the controls. Both groups showed highly significant improvements in extension but straight leg raising improved significantly only in the active treatment group.

At 3 months symptoms did not differ between the two groups. Objective measurements showed no change in spinal flexion in those who had received active treatment but the significant deterioration in the controls was maintained. Both groups still showed significant improvement in extension. The patients who received mobilization showed slightly greater overall improvements than the controls but the differences seen at 1 month had largely disappeared. At 1 year symptoms were similar in the two groups.

The presenting features were compared in the one-third patients who did best and the one-third patients who did worst immediately after treatment. The only prognostic factor to emerge was that patients with pain duration of less than a month more frequently improved than those with a history of longer than a month. This enhanced effect in patients with short histories was also seen both in the trials of Glover, Morris and Khosla and Evans et al. Sims-Williams et al. noted that their patients may not have had as severe disease as those attending hospital, and hospital patients would probably not show such a high rate of improvement. The authors concluded that most sufferers from back pain obtain relief without any specific treatment but mobilization and manipulation may hasten this improvement without making any difference to the long-term prognosis.

Manipulation hastened improvement in all of the clinical trials irrespective of the technique used. Similarly there was never any effect in the long term. Jayson (personal communication) has used the analogy of back pain persuing a relapsing and remitting course analagous to that of chronic bronchitis. Courses of antibiotics may help to relieve acute attacks of the latter, although they may make no difference in the long term. It may be that repeated courses of manipulation will be helpful to some patients in providing a longer-term control in the same way as repeated courses of antibiotics, but this remains to be determined. Some practitioners advocate regular manipulative treatments three or four times in a year to anticipate and prevent a recurrent attack. Of special interest is the increased response found by Evans *et al.* in patients over 45 years of age. This is the age when segmental instability secondary to previous disc or ligamentous disease leads to subluxation of the facet joints. I would not argue with the term 'locking' of the facet joints instead of subluxation as the former may only be an extreme case of the latter. The subluxation is a mechanical pathological entity that responds to a mechanical solution. This mechanism also explains why it is those patients with relatively short histories who improve the most. These *are* the patients with acute-on-chronic low back pain which is a manifestation of facet joint subluxation. They improve spontaneously anyway given time, but manipulation may reduce the subluxation which often is being maintained by superimposed muscle spasm.

Mathews and Yates (1969) postulate a different mechanism for the relief of symptoms of mechanical lumbar spine disorder by manipulation. They incriminated small disc prolapses in two patients and were able to show by epidurography both the presence of these pretreatment and a reduction in size of the lesions after manipulation. Both patients had pain of rapid onset which was of less than a week's duration when treated. The first case, a woman aged 45 years, had a history and signs suggestive of an acute disc prolapse so it was not surprising that the epidurograph showed a lesion in the region of the L_4-L_5 disc. Immediately afterwards but before manipulation, the pain disappeared and the straight-leg-raising test returned to normal so the role that subsequent manipulation played is difficult to discern. The second case, a man of 45, had suffered many previous attacks and, despite his borderline age, his history fits well into my subluxation group. I would expect him to derive benefit from manipulation, as he indeed did. Reductions of concavities over the discs as shown by epidurographs were presented by the authors as reductions in disc protrusions and they showed similar changes in a further three cases. Thus one must accept the possibility that *small* disc protrusions can be reduced by manipulation. Chrisman, Mittnacht and Snook (1964) failed to show any reduction in the size of larger and more lateral protrusions following manipulation. Further patients of these investigators with normal myelograms fared rather better with manipulation and it may be that these fell into the 'facet-joint − subluxation' category.

Bearing in mind these two possible mechanisms of action, when should manipulation be attempted? Certainly for patients aged 45 years or more with repeated attacks of low back pain, manipulation is the treatment of choice. It is simple, quick, painfree and, if practised by trained and qualified therapists, safe. Adverse events are reported in the literature but they are rare and can largely be avoided. In younger patients, particularly those suspected of having *small* disc prolapses or premature segmental instability secondary to disc disease (and rarely to ligamentous stretching), manipulation is worth attempting. It is contraindicated where gross neurological signs are present and should usually be avoided in the hypermobile patient.

Manipulation restores normal mobility and is indicated when there is some restriction of movement. Doran and Newell suggested that manipulation is more effective in those cases with painful limitation of extension. Sims-Williams *et al.* found significant improvements in extension not only in their treated group but also in their control group. The difference between groups (at 1 and 3 months) lay in spinal flexion. The patients in the manipulated group showed no change in flexion whereas those in the control group exhibited a significant deterioration compared to their starting value. In the trial of Evans *et al.* spinal flexion increased significantly in the manipulated group in the 3 weeks of treatment but there was a significant decrease in the 3-week period after manipulation. Therefore it seems that spinal flexion is a very labile parameter which deteriorates during periods of low back pain. This deterioration can be prevented, and during courses of treatment reversed, by manipulation. Spinal extension seems to improve irrespective of the type of treatment given.

The various techniques are described well by Bourdillon (1973), Cyriax (1971) and Maitland (1977) and will not be described here. As a general rule rotational manipulation has been shown to give the best results whereas symptoms are sometimes worsened by anteroposterior lumbar manipulation. Rotational lumbar manipulation is not the instant, magical cure it is often made out to be. For a couple of days after treatment the patient usually suffers more pain than that present before the procedure. The original symptoms are back by the end of the first week when the second manipulation is administered. In suitable cases improvement then proceeds quickly and only rarely is a third treatment necessary. Because the type of low back pain that responds to manipulation is a recurrent condition, further manipulations are often necessary 4−6 months later and subsequent attacks can sometimes be prevented if treatment is prescribed routinely at 4−6-month intervals.

IN SUMMARY

132.   Spinal manipulation refers to many different forms of treatment but in Britain there are two common types. The one predominantly referred to in this chapter is a rotational thrust with distraction consisting of small-amplitude, high-velocity movements. This is performed without an anaesthetic, as is the second type which consists of repetitive, gentle, oscillatory movements often called mobilizations.

133.   Although this form of treatment is one of the most emotive in modern medicine, it is gaining orthodox acceptance since the publication of controlled clinical trials, which have been conducted by:

(1) Glover, Morris, and Khosla (1974)
(2) Doran and Newell (1975)
(3) Evans et al. (1978)
(4) Sims-Williams et al. (1978)

134.   Methodology of these trials included:

Trial	Type of manipulation	Control	Duration of assessments	Special features
(1)	rotational	detuned shortwave diathermy	1 month	unilateral pain only
(2)	various	physio-therapy, corsets, analgesics	1 year	multicentre
(3)	rotational	analgesics	6 weeks	crossover
(4)	mobilization	placebo microwave	1 year	general practice patients

135.   The conclusions of these trials were:

A – manipulation hastened improvement   Trial
more pain relief in treated group immediately after manipul-   (1)
ation
more manipulated patients reported improvement at   (2)
3 weeks
less pain in second and third week after treatment in man-   (3)
ipulated group
pain scores reduced significantly only in manipulated group   (3)
reduced pain at 1 month more common in manipulation   (4)
group

B – no effect in long-term
at 6 weeks and thereafter no difference between groups   (2)
at 3 months and thereafter no difference between groups   (4)
C – better response in older patients
responders significantly older than non-responders   (3)
D – better response associated with short history
patients with less than 1 week's history improved more rapidly (1)
than those with longer history
duration of back pain shorter in responders   (3)
patients with less than 1 month's history fared better than   (4)
those with longer history
E – first week of treatment with manipulation painful
first week after manipulation more painful than correspond- (1) and
ing first week after control   (3)
F – increase in spinal flexion associated with manipulation
significant increase in manipulated group   (3)
deterioration only in control group   (4)
G – increase in spinal extension associated with both treat- (4)
ments
H – radiography contributes little except to exclude serious (3)
pathology

136.   These conclusions were used to postulate:
A – spinal manipulation reduces subluxation or frees locking of facet joints in patients with segmental instability secondary to previous disc or ligamentous disease.
B – these patients tend to be 45 years old or more and suffer from recurrent attacks of acute-on-chronic backache. They improve spontaneously given time but spinal manipulation may hasten improvement by reducing the subluxation which is being maintained by superimposed muscle spasm.

137.   Mathews and Yates (1969) describe reduction of *small* disc prolapses by manipulation and provide good evidence for the existence of this alternative indication for this treatment.

138.   Manipulation is therefore:
A – the treatment of choice in patients of 45 years of age or more with recurrent attacks of low back pain.
B – worth attempting in younger patients suspected of having a *small* disc prolapse
C – contraindicated where gross neurological signs are present
D – usually to be avoided in the hypermobile patient
E – indicated where there is some restriction of spinal movement
F – useful in regular treatments every 4–6 months to prevent subsequent attacks.

References and further reading

Adams, J.C. (1971). *Outline of Orthopaedics*. (Edinburgh: Churchill Livingstone)

Akerblom, B. (1948). *Standing and Sitting Posture*. (Stockholm: A-B Nordiska Bokhandeln)

Andersson, S.A., Hansson, G., Holmgren, E. and Renberg, O. (1976). Evaluation of the pain suppressive effect of different frequencies of peripheral electrical stimulation in chronic pain conditions. *Acta Orthop. Scand.*, **47**, 149–57

Anonymous. (1978). Apophyseal joints and back pain. *Lancet*, **2**, 247

Asmussen, E. and Heebøll-Nielsen, K. (1959). Posture, mobility and strength of the back in boys, 7 to 16 years old. *Acta Orthop. Scand.*, **28**, 174–189

Asmussen, E. and Klausen, K. (1962). Form and function of the erect human spine. *Clin. Orthop.*, **25**, 55–63

Attenborough, D. (1979). *Life on Earth*. (London: BBC/Collins)

Baddeley, H. (1976). Radiology of lumbar spinal stenosis. In Jayson, M.I.V. (ed.) *The Lumbar Spine and Back Pain*. pp. 151–171. (London: Sector Publishing)

Ballesteros, M.L.F. *et al.* (1965). The pattern of muscular activity during the arm swing of natural walking. *Acta Physiol. Scand.*, **63**, 296–310

Bartelink, D.L. (1957). The role of abdominal pressure in relieving the pressure on the lumbar intervertebral discs. *J. Bone Jt. Surg. [Br.]*, **39**, 718–25

Basmajian, J.V. (1958). Electromyography of iliopsoas. *Anat. Rec.*, **132**, 127–132

Beadle, O.A. (1931). The intervertebral disc. *Medical Council Special Report No. 161*. London

Beck, A. and Killus, J. (1973). Normal posture of spine determined by mathematical and statistical methods. *Aerospace Med.*, **41**(11), 1277–81

Beetham, W.P., Polley, H.F., Slocumb, C.H. and Weaver, W.F. (1966). *Physical Examination of the Joints*. (Philadelphia: W.B. Saunders)

Belenky, V.E. (1971). Study of the movements of the pelvis and spine during walking. *Ortop. Travmatol. Protez.*, **32**, 37–43

Beliveau, P. (1971). A comparison between epidural anaesthesia with and without corticosteroid in the treatment of sciatica. *Rheum. Phys. Med.*, **11**, 40–3

Blight, A.R. (1976). Undulatory swimming with and without waves of contraction. *Nature (London)*, **264**(5584), 352–4

Bourdillon J.F. (1973). *Spinal manipulation.* 2nd edn. (London: Heinemann Medical)

Bourne, I.H.J. (1979). Treatment of backache with local injections. *Practitioner,* **222,** 708–11

Brish, A., Lerner, M.A. and Braham, J. (1964). Intermittent claudication from compression of cauda equina by a narrowed spinal canal. *J. Neurosurg.,* **21,** 207–11

Chabot, J. (1962). *Les Consultations Journalières en Rhumatologie.* (Paris: Masson)

Chrisman, O.D., Mittnacht, A. and Snook, G.A. (1964). A study of the results following rotatory manipulation in the lumbar intervertebral-disc syndrome. *J. Bone Jt. Surg.,* **46A,** 517

Ciocci, A. (1976). Indomethacin in the treatment of the lumbar disc syndrome. In Huskisson, E.C. and Velo, G.P. (eds.) *Inflammatory Arthropathies.* pp. 179–83. (Amsterdam: Excerpta Medica)

Close, J.R. (1964). *Motor Function in the Lower Extremity.* (Springfield: Charles C. Thomas)

Coomes, E.N. (1961). A comparison between epidural anaesthesia and bed rest in sciatica. *Br. Med. J.,* **1,** 20–4

Coplans, C.W. (1978). The conservative treatment of low back pain. In Helfet, A.J. and Lee, D.M.G. (eds.) *Disorder of the Lumbar Spine.* pp. 145–183. (Philadelphia: J.B. Lippincott)

Coxhead, C.E. (1974). A clinical trial of the management of sciatica with or without low back pain. *Physiotherapy,* **60,** 72–4

Cyriax, J. (1969). *Textbook of Orthopaedic Medicine.* Vol. 1, 5th edn. (London: Baillière Tindall and Cassell)

Cyriax, J. (1971). *Textbook of Orthopaedic Medicine.* Vol. 2, 8th edn. (London: Baillière Tindall and Cassell)

Davis, P. and Lentle, B.C. (1978). Evidence for sacroiliac disease as a common cause of low backache in women. *Lancet,* **2,** 496–7

Davis, P.R. (1968). On being upright. In: Passmore, R. and Robson, J.S. (eds.) *A Companion to Medical Studies.* Vol. 1, 46.1–46.2. (Oxford: Blackwell Scientific Publications)

Davis, P.R. (1959). The medial inclincation of the human thoracic intervertebral articular facets. *J. Anat.,* **93,** 68–74

Dehlin, O., Berg, S., Hedenrud, B., Andersson, G. and Grimby, G. (1978). Muscle training, psychological perception of work and low-back symptoms in nursing aides. *Scand. J. Rehab. Med.,* **10,** 201–9

Delmas, A. (Cited in Kapandji, 1974)

De Roo, M., Walravens, M. and Dequeker, J. (1978). Sacroiliac disease and low backache in women. *Lancet,* **2,** 942–3

De Seze (Cited in Kapandji, 1974)

Dilke, T.F.W., Burry, H.C. and Grahame, R. (1973). Extradural corticosteroid injection in management of lumbar nerve root compression. *Br. Med. J.,* **2,** 635–7

Dixon, A. St J. (1976). Foreword. In Jayson, M.I.V. (ed.) *The Lumbar Spine and Back Pain.* pp. 7–11. (London: Sector Publishing)

Doran, D.M.L. and Newell, D.J. (1975). Manipulation in treatment of low back pain: A multicentre study. *Br. Med. J.,* **2,** 161–4

Dougherty, J.H. and Fraser, R.A.R. (1978). Complications following intraspinal injections of steroids. Report of two cases. *J. Neurosurg.,* **48,** 1023–5

Duncan, D.B. (1955). Multiple range and multiple F tests. *Biometrics,* **11,** 1–42

Edelist, G., Gross, A.E. and Langer, F. (1976). Treatment of low back pain with acupuncture. *Can. Anaesth. Soc. J.,* **23(3),** 303–6

Eie, N. and Wehn, P. (1962). Measurements of the intra-abdominal pressure in relation to weightbearing of the lumbosacral spine. *J. Oslo City Hosp.,* **12,** 205–17

Eiseley, L.C. (1953). Fossil man. *Sci. Am.*, **189**, 65–72

Ellis, J. (1944). Compression fractures of vertebral bodies. *J. Bone Jt. Surg.*, **42**, 139

Evans, D.P., Burke, M.S., Lloyd, K.N., Roberts, E.E. and Roberts, G.M. (1978). Lumbar spinal manipulation on trial. Part 1 – clinical assessment. *Rheum. Rehabil.*, **17**, 46–53

Evans D.P. (1980). Extended-heel shoes. *Rheum. Rehabil.*, **19**, 103–8

Evans D.P., Burke, M.S. and Newcombe, R.G. (1980). Medicines of choice in low back pain. *Curr. Med. Res. Opin.*, **6**, 540–7

Evans F. G. (1946). The anatomy and function of the foreleg in salamander locomotion. *Anat. Rec.*, **95**, 257–81

Farfan, H.F. and Sullivan, J.D. (1967). The relation of facet orientation to intervertebral disc failure. *Can. J. Surg.*, **10**, 179–85

Farfan, H.F., Cossette, J.W., Robertson, G.H., Wells, R.V. and Kraus, H. (1970). The effects of torsion on the lumbar intervertebral joints: The role of torsion in the production of disc degeneration. *J. Bone Jt. Surg.*, **52A**, 468–97

Farfan, H.F. (1973). *Mechanical Disorders of the Low Back.* (Philadelphia: Lea and Febiger)

Farfan, H.F. (1978). The biomechanical advantage of lordosis and hip extension for upright activity. *Spine*, **3**, 336–42

Farfan, H.F. and Sullivan, J.D. (1967). The relation of facet orientation to intervertebral disc failure. *Can. J. Surg.*, **10**, 179–85

Farfan, H.F. (1969). The effects of torsion on the intervertebral joints. *Can. J. Surg.*, **12**, 336–41

Floyd, W.F. and Silver, P.H.S. (1950). Electromyographic study of patterns of activity of the anterior abdominal wall muscles in man. *J. Anat.*, **84**, 132

Fox, E.J. and Melzack, R. (1976). Transcutaneous electrical stimulation and acupuncture: comparison of treatment for low-back pain. *Pain*, **2**, 141–8

Glover, J.R., Morris, J.G. and Khosla, T. (1974). Back pain: a randomized clinical trial of rotational manipulation of the trunk. *Br. J. Ind. Med.*, **31**, 59–64

Goff, C.W. (1952). Orthograms of posture. *J. Bone Jt. Surg.*, **34A**, 115

Goldie, I. (1968). A clinical trial with indomethacin (Indomee) in low back pain and sciatica. *Acta Orthop. Scand.*, **39**, 117–28

Gray, H. (1973). *Gray's Anatomy.* 35th edn., Warwick, R. and Williams, P.L. (eds.) p. 111. (Edinburgh: Longman)

Gray, J. (1944). Studies in the mechanics of the tetrapod skeleton. *J. Exp. Biol.*, **20**, 88–116

Gray, J. (1959). *How Animals Move.* (Harmondsworth: Penguin)

Gregersen, G.G. and Lucas, D.B. (1967). An in vivo study of the axial rotation of the human thoracolumbar spine. *J. Bone Jt. Surg.*, **49A**, 247–262

Grevsten, S. and Johansson, H. (1975). Phenylbutazone in treatment of acute lumbago-sciatica. *Z. Rheumatol.*, **34**, 444–7

Harris, R.I. and Macnab, I. (1954). Structural changes in the lumbar intervertebral discs. *J. Bone Jt. Surg.*, **36B**, 304

Hart, F.D. (1978). *Drug Treatment of the Rheumatic Diseases.* (Lancaster: MTP Press)

Hawkes, C.H. and Roberts, G.M. (1980). Lumbar canal stenosis. *Br. J. Hosp. Med.*, **23**, 498–505

Helfet, A.J. and Lee, D.M.G. (1978). *Disorders of the Lumbar Spine.* (Philadelphia: J.B. Lippincott)

Hingorani, K. and Templeton, J.S. (1975). A comparative trial of azapropazone and ketoprofen in the treatment of acute backache. *Curr. Med. Res. Opin.*, **3**, 407–12

Hingorani, K. (1971). Orphenadrine/paracetamol in backache – a double-blind controlled trial. *Br. J. Clin. Pract.*, **25**, 227–31

Hingorani, K. and Biswas, A.K. (1970). Double-blind controlled trial comparing oxyphenbutazone and indomethacin in the treatment of acute low back pain. *Br. J. Clin. Pract.*, **24**, 120–3

Hingorani, K. (1966). Diazepam in backache, A double-blind controlled trial. *Ann. Phys. Med.*, **8**, 303–6

Hirsch, C. and Nachemson, A. (1954). New observations on the mechanical behaviour of lumbar discs. *Acta Orthop. Scand.*, **23**, 254–83

Hirsch, C. and Nachemson, A. (1961). Clinical observations on the spine in ejected pilots. *Acta Orthop. Scand.*, **31**, 135

Hirsch, C.J., Jonsson, B. and Lewin, T. (1969). Low-back symptoms in a Swedish female population. *Clin. Orthop.*, **63**, 171–6

Howes, R.J. and Isdale, I.C. (1971). The loose back: an unrecognized syndrome. *Rheum. Phys. Med.*, **11**, 72–7

Isdale, I.C. personal communication to Moll, J. and Wright, V. (1976). Measurement of spinal movement. In Jayson, M.I.V. (ed.) *The Lumbar Spine and Back Pain*, (London: Sector Publishing)

Jacobs, J.H. and Grayson, M.F. (1968). Trial of an anti-inflammatory agent (indomethacin) in low back pain with and without radicular involvement. *Br. Med. J.*, **3**, 158–60

Jaffé, G. (1974). A double-blind, between-patient comparison of alclofenac ('Prinalgin') and indomethacin in the treatment of low back pain and sciatica. *Curr. Med. Res. Opin.*, **2**, 424–9

Jamiolkowska, K. (1973). Planes and axes of rotation of the vertebral column in man. *Folia Morphol. (Warsz.)*, **32**, 371–9

Jayson, M.I.V. Personal communication

Jayson, M.I.V. and Nelson, M.A. (1979). Spinal stenosis and low back pain. *Reports on rheumatic diseases 1979, No. 70* (London: The Arthritis and Rheumatism Council)

Jayson, M.I.V. (1978). Back pain, spondylosis and disc disorders. In Scott, J.T. (ed.) *Copeman's Textbook of the Rheumatic Diseases*, pp. 960–85. (Edinburgh: Churchill Livingstone)

Jenkins, D.G., Ebbutt, A.F. and Evans, C.D. (1976). Tofranil in the treatment of low back pain. *J. Int. Med. Res.*, **4**, Suppl. 2, 28–40

Jenni, D.A. and Jenni, M.A. (1976). Carrying behaviour in humans: analysis of sex differences. *Science*, **194**, 859–60

Joseph, J. (1960). *Man's Posture: Electromyographic Studies.* (Springfield: Charles C. Thomas)

Kapandji, I.A. (1974). *The Physiology of the Joints.* Vol. 3. (Edinburgh: Churchill Livingstone)

Keith, A. (1923). Man's posture: its evolution and disorders. *Br. Med. J.*, **1**, 451–4; 499–502; 545–8; 587–90; 624–6 and 669–72

Kellgren, J.H. (1978). Pain. In Scott, J.T. (ed.) *Copeman's Textbook of the Rheumatic Diseases.* 5th edn. (Edinburgh: Churchill Livingstone)

Kendall, P.H. and Jenkins, J.M. (1968). Exercises for backache; A double-blind controlled trial. *Physiotherapy*, **54**, 154–7

Kent, G.C. (1973). *Comparative Anatomy of the Vertebrates.* (St Louis: C.V. Mosby)

Krogman, W.M. (1962). Man's posture. Where from? Where to? *Clin. Orthop.*, **25**, 98–109

Laitinen, J. (1976). Acupuncture and transcutaneous electric stimulation in the treatment of chronic sacrolumbalgia and ischialgia. *Am. J. Chin. Med.*, **4**, 169–75

Lange, C. (1902). Untersuchungen über Elasticitäts Verhältnisse in den menschlichen Rückenwirzblen mit Bermerkungen über die Pathogenese der Deformatäten. *Z. Orthop. Chir.*, **10**, 47

Laurell, L. and Nachemson, A. (1961). Some factors influencing spine injuries in seat ejected pilots. *Rev. Med. Aero(Paris)*, **2**, 195–6

Lawrence, J.S., Bremner, J.M. and Bier, F. (1966). Osteoarthrosis: prevalence in the population and relationship between symptoms and x-ray changes. *Ann. Rheum. Dis.*, **25**, 1

Le Gros Clark, W.E. (1955). *Fossil Evidence for Human Evolution*. (Chicago: University of Chicago Press)

Leger, W. (1968). Die Wirbelsäulenhaltung und ihre krankhaften Störungen. *Wochenschr. Forsch. Praxis*, **40**, 25–34

Lidström, A. and Zachrisson, M. (1970). Physical therapy on low back pain and sciatica. *Scand. J. Rehab. Med.*, **2**, 37–42

Loebl, W.Y. (1973). Regional rotation of the spine. *Rheumatol. Rehab.*, **12**, 223

Lovejoy, C.O., Heiple, K.G. and Burstein, A.H. (1973). The gait of Australopitheca. *Am. J. Phys. Anthrop.*, **38**, 757–80

Lucas, D.B. and Bresler, B. (1961). Stability of the ligamentous spine. *Technical report No. 40. San Francisco, Biomechanics Laboratory,* University of California

Lucas, D.B. (1970). Mechanics of the spine. *Bull. Hosp. Joint. Dis.*, **31**(2), 115–131

Macnab, I. (1977). *Backache*. (Baltimore: Williams & Wilkins)

Maitland, G.D. (1977). *Vertebral Manipulation*. 4th edn. (London: Butterworths)

Mark, L.C. (1973). Double-blind studies of acupuncture. *J. Am. Med. Assoc.*, **225**, 1532

Markolf, K.L. (1972). Deformation of the thoracolumbar intervertebral joints in response to external loads. *J. Bone Jt. Surg.*, **54A**, 511–33

Martin, R. (1977). Man is not an onion. *New Sci.*, **75**(1063), 283–5

Maslow, G.S. and Rothman R. (1975). The facet joints: another look. *Bull. NY Acad. Med.*, **51**(11), 1294–1311

Mathews, J.A. and Yates, D.A.H. (1969). Reduction of lumbar disc prolapse by manipulation. *Br. Med. J.*, **3**, 696–7

McHenry, H.M. and Corruccini, R.S. (1976). Fossil hominid femora and the evolution of walking. *Nature (Lond.)*, **259**, 657–8

Mckenzie, R.A. (1979). Prophylaxis in recurrent low back pain. *NZ Med. J.*, **89**, 22–3

Mednick, L.W. (1955). The evolution of the human ilium. *Am. J. Phys. Anthrop.*, **13**(2), 203–216

Melzack, R. (1975). Prolonged relief of pain by brief, intense transcutaneous somatic stimulation. *Pain*, **1**, 357–73

Melzack, R. (1973). *The Puzzle of Pain*. (Harmondsworth: Penguin Books)

Mendelson, G, Kranz, H., Kidson, M.A., Loh, S.T., Scott, D.F. and Selwood T.S. (1977). Acupuncture for chronic back pain: patients and methods. *Proc. Aust. Assoc. Neurol.*, **14**, 154–61

Messerer, O. (1880). *Uber Elasticität und Festigkeit der Menschlichen Knochen.* Stuttgart

Moll, J.M.H. and Wright, V. (1971). Normal range of spinal mobility: an objective clinical study. *Ann. Rheum. Dis.*, **30**, 381–6

Mooney, V. and Robertson, J. (1976). The facet syndrome. *Clin. Orthop.*, **115**, 149–56

Morris, J.M., Lucas, D.B. and Bresler, B. (1961). Role of the trunk in stability of the spine. *J. Bone Jt. Surg.*, **43**, 327–51

Morris, J.M. (1973). Biomechanics of the spine. *Arch. Surg.*, **107**, 418–23

Nachemson, A. (1962). Some mechanical properties of the lumbar intervertebral discs. *Bull. Hosp. Jt. Dis.*, **23**, 130–43

Nachemson, A. (1976). Lumbar intradiscal pressure. In Jayson, M.I.V. (ed.) *The lumbar Spine and Back Pain.* pp. 257–69. (London: Sector Publishing)

Nachemson, A. (1976). A critical look at conservative treatment for low back pain. In Jayson, M.I.V. (ed.) *The Lumbar Spine and Back Pain.* pp. 355–65. (London: Sector Publishing)

Nachemson, A. (1960). Lumbar intradiscal pressure. *Acta Orthop. Scand.,* Suppl. 43, 1–104

Nachemson, A. (1976). The lumbar spine. An orthopedic challenge. *Spine,* **1**, 59–71

Nachemson, A. (1966). EMG studies on the vertebral portion of the psoas muscle. *Acta Orthop. Scand.,* **37**, 177

Nachemson, A. and Evans, J. (1968). Some mechanical properties of the third human lumbar interlaminar ligament (ligamentum flavum). *J. Biomechanics,* **1**, 211

Napier, J. (1967). The antiquity of human walking. *Sci. Am.,* **216**, 56–66

Perey, O. (1957). Fracture of the vertebral end-plate in the lumbar spine. An experimental biomechanical investigation. *Acta Orthop. Scand.,* Suppl. 25

Petersen, K. (1963). *Prehistoric Life on Earth.* (London: Methuen)

Pickford, M. (1977). Pre-human fossils from Pakistan. *New Sci.,* **75**(1068), 578–80

Pitkin, H.C. and Pheasant, H.C. (1936). Sacrarthrogenic telalgia. *J. Bone Jt. Surg.,* **18**, 111–133; 365–74

Roaf, R. (1960). A study of mechanics of spinal injury. *J. Bone Jt. Surg.,* **42B**, 810

Roaf, R. (1977). *Posture.* (London: Academic Press)

Roberts, G.M. (1978). MD thesis. University of London

Roberts, G.M., Roberts, E.E., Lloyd, K.N., Burke, M.S. and Evans, D.P. (1978). Lumbar spinal manipulation on trial. Part II – radiological assessment. *Rheum. Rehabil.,* **17**, 54–9

Romer, A.S. (1960). *Man and the Vertebrates.* Vol. 1 and 2. (Harmondsworth: Penguin)

Ruff, S. (1945). Human tolerance to acceleration. In *German Aviation Medicine, World War II.* Washington DC, 584

Sayle-Creer, W. and Swerdlow, M. (1969). Epidural injections for the relief of lumbosciatic pain. *Acta Orthop. Belg.,* **35**, 728–34

Schiötz, E. and Cyriax, J. (1975). *Manipulation past and present.* (London: Heinemann)

Schmorl, G. and Junghanns, H. (1971). *The Human Spine in Health and Disease.* (Transl. Besemann, E.F.) (New York and London: Grune and Stratton)

Schmorl, G. (1926). Die Pathologische Anatomie der Wirbersaule. *Verh. Dtsch. Orthop. Ges.,* **21**, 3

Schultz, A.H. (1950). The specializations of man and his place among the catarrhine primates. In Demerec, M. (ed.) *Origin and Evolution of Man. Symposia Quant. Biol.,* **15**, 37–53

Scott, G.L., Myles, A.B. and Bacon, P.A. (1968). Autoimmune haemolytic anaemia and mefenamic acid therapy. *Br. Med. J.,* **3**, 534–5

Shah, J.S., Coggins, J., Rogers, R., Jayson, M.I.V. and Hampson, W.G.J. (1976). Surface strain distribution in isolated single lumbar vertebrae. *Ann. Rheum. Dis.,* **35**, 51–55

Shah, J.S. (1976). Experimental stress analysis of the lumbar spine. In Jayson, M.I.V. (ed.) *The Lumbar Spine and Back Pain.* pp. 271–292. (London: Sector Publishing)

Sharma, R.K. (1977). Indications, technique and results of caudal epidural injection for lumbar disc retropulsion. *Postgrad. Med. J.,* **53**, 1–6

Simons, E.L. (1977). Ramapithecus. *Sci. Am.,* **236**, 28–35

Sims-Williams, H., Jayson, M.I.V., Young, S.M.S., Baddeley, H. and Collins, E. (1978). Controlled trial of mobilization and manipulation for patients with low back pain in general practice. *Br. Med. J.,* **2**, 1338–40

Sims-Williams, H,. Jayson, M.I.V., Baddeley, H. (1978). Small spinal fractures in back pain patients. *Ann. Rheum. Dis.,* **37**, 262–265

Snijders, I.C.J. (1969). On the form of the human spine and some aspects of its mechanical behaviour. *Acta Orthop. Belg.*, **35**, 584–94

Staffel, F. (1889). *Die menschlichen Haltungstypen und ihre Beziehungen zu den Rückratsverkrümmungen.* Wiesbaden

Steindler, A. (1955). *Kinesiology of the Human body, 2nd edn.* (Springfield: Charles C. Thomas)

Stillwell, G.K. (1973). The law of Laplace. Some clinical applications. *Mayo Clin. Proc.*, **48**, 863–9

Straus, W.L. (1962). Fossil evidence of the evolution of the erect, bipedal posture. *Clin. Orthop.*, **25**, 9–19

Sturrock, R.D., Wojtulewski, J.A. and Hart, F.D. (1973). Spondylometry in a normal population and in ankylosing spondylitis. *Rheumatol. Rehab.*, **12**, 135–42

Tanz, S.S. (1953). Motion of the lumbar spine. A roentgenologic study. *Am. J. Roentgenol.*, **69**, 399–412

Tanz, S.S. (1950). To-and-fro motion range at the fourth and fifth lumbar interspaces. *J. Mt. Sinai Hosp.*, **16**, 303–307

Thompson, d'A.W. (1942). *On Growth and Form.* (Cambridge: Cambridge University Press)

Travell, J. and Rinzler, S.H. (1952). The myofascial genesis of pain. *Postgrad. Med.*, **11**, 425–34

Vernon-Roberts, B. (1976). Pathology of degenerative spondylosis. In Jayson, M.I.V. (ed.) *The Lumbar Spine and Back Pain.* pp. 55–75. (London: Sector Publishing)

Virgin, W.J. (1951). Experimental investigations into the physical properties of the intervertebral disc. *J. Bone Jt. Surg.*, **33B**, 607

Washburn, S.L. (1960). Tools and human evolution. *Sci. Am.*, **203**, 63–75

Weisl, H. (1955). Movement of the sacroiliac joint. *Acta Anat.*, **23**, 80–91

White, A.A. and Hirsch, C. (1971). The significance of the vertebral posterior elements in the mechanics of the thoracic spine. *Clin. Orthop. Rel. Res.*, **81**, 2–14

Wilber, M.C. (1975). Sedation of active acupuncture loci in the management of low back pain. *Am. J. Chin. Med.*, **3**, 275–9

Williams, P.C. (1974). *Low Back and Neck Pain: Causes and Conservative Treatment.* (Springfield: Charles C. Thomas)

Wiltse, L.L., Widdell, E.H. and Jackson, D.W. (1975). Fatigue fracture: the basic lesion in isthmic spondylolisthesis. *J. Bone Jt. Surg.*, **57A**, 17–22

Wood, P.H.N. (1976). Epidemiology of back pain. In Jayson, M.I.V. (ed.) *The lumbar Spine and Back Pain.* pp. 13–27. (London: Sector Publishing)

Working Group on Back Pain. (1979). *Report to Secretary of State for Social Services, Secretary of State for Scotland.* (London: HMSO)

Wyke, B. (1976). Neurological aspects of low back pain. In Jayson, M.I.V. (ed.) *The Lumbar Spine and Back Pain.* pp. 189–256. (London: Sector Publishing)

Yamada, K. (1962). The dynamics of experimental posture. *Clin. Orthop.*, **25**, 20–31

Yates, D.W. (1978). A comparison of the types of epidural injection commonly used in the treatment of low back pain and sciatica. *Rheum. Rehab.*, **17**, 181–6

Young, J.Z. (1975). *The Life of Mammals: their Anatomy and Physiology.* (Oxford: Clarendon Press)

Index